The Biology of the Brain

The Biology of the Brain
From Neurons to Networks

· · ·

READINGS FROM
SCIENTIFIC AMERICAN
MAGAZINE

Edited by

Rodolfo R. Llinás
New York University Medical Center

W. H. FREEMAN AND COMPANY
New York

Some of the SCIENTIFIC AMERICAN articles in *The Biology of the Brain: From Neurons to Networks* are available as separate Offprints. For a complete list of articles now available as Offprints, write to W. H. Freeman and Company, 41 Madison Avenue, New York, New York 10010.

Library of Congress Cataloging-in-Publication Data

The Biology of the brain.

   Collection of articles previously published in Scientific American, 1977–1988.
   Bibliography: p.
   Includes index.
   1. Brain.   2. Neurophysiology.   I. Llinás,
Rodolfo R. (Rodolfo Riascos), 1934–   II. Scientific American.
[DNLM: 1. Brain—physiology—collected works.
2. Neurobiology—collected works. WL 300 B6156]
QP376.B623   1989   612'.82   88-36263
ISBN 0-7167-2037-X

Printed in the United States of America

1234567890 RRD 7654321089

CONTENTS

Note on cross-references to SCIENTIFIC AMERICAN *articles*: Articles included in this book are referred to by chapter number and title; articles not included in this book but available as Offprints are referred to by title, date of publication, and Offprint number; articles not in this book and not available as Offprints are referred to by title and date of publication.

Introduction

Neuroscience has experienced an explosive development over the past fifteen years. An unprecedented increase of knowledge and the variety and power of the new techniques of study have served as the impetus for assembling this book. Among the significant events of this period in neuroscience has been the realization that understanding the workings of the brain requires a multidisciplinary approach. Thus, neuroscience has been released from the constraints of particular sets of techniques and disciplines and has become one of the most impressive and promising areas of biological and theoretical research. Central to this new approach is the realization of the importance of detailed, quantitative understanding of the basic biophysical and biochemical machinery comprising the molecular constituents of nerve cells. The results gathered during this period represent basic knowledge about the functioning of the nervous system on all levels of evolution.

The central theme of this book reflects the view that, as far as we can tell today, the brain, as complex as it is, can only be understood from a cellular perspective. This perspective has been the cornerstone of neuroscience over the past 100 years. Historically, the question of the relation of the body to the mind was, at best, opaque; the mental attributes of humans were only vaguely related to the attributes of the brain. Despite the increase in our knowledge of brain morphology and function at the end of the nineteenth century and the beginning of the twentieth century, there was still a feeling among many scholars that the nature of human reason might be related to some new and wonderful knowledge totally alien to that which is accessible through the scientific method.

The battle to reduce brain function to that of a "society" of interconnected cellular elements was won with the "neuron doctrine," presented in its clearest form by Ramón y Cajal in 1933. This doctrine proposed that the brain is not an amorphous mass of tissue in which every part is related to every other in a spiderweb fashion, but rather is an exquisitely organized society of totally separate nerve cells. Moreover, this doctrine, which is universally accepted today, states that every individual neuron has a particular function and form and, most importantly, a particular set of connections to other neurons. Accordingly, only when the brain was seen to be a cellular society where each element integrates information individually did the complexity of the brain machinery begin to emerge.

Today, while many neuroscientists suspect that understanding the mind means understanding the properties of sensory motor transformations that ultimately rule brain function, others adhere to the dualist view that mind and brain are separate entities. Regardless of one's view, the fact remains that the scientific method is our only tool in the struggle for knowledge and understanding. Thus, the chapters in *The Biology of the Brain* tell the story of some attempts by scientists to comprehend the nature of the brain and its function by studying the properties of individual cellular elements.

The Neuron

If the brain is a cellular ensemble, its function must be inscribed in the properties of neurons and their synaptic connectivity—that is, in the spontaneous electrical activity of individual neurons derived directly from their intrinsic membrane properties and their connectivity with other neurons. According to this view, the functional properties of the brain arise not merely from the information transmitted by pathways from cell to cell, but also from the specific intrinsic properties of each of the neuronal elements in the transmission chain.

Chapter 1, "The Neuron," by Charles F. Stevens, reviews the functional aspects of individual neurons. Stevens discusses in some detail the properties of the protein molecules that traverse the external surface membrane of the cell and how this protein links the inside of the cell with its extracellular environment. Among other functions, these large protein molecules allow ions to move across the membrane and thus generate ionic currents. The role of the various membrane-specific components in cell communication through the genesis of the so-called action potential (the nerve impulse) and synaptic-transmitter release is also discussed as molecular biology is brought into the context of neuron physiology.

Communication between Neurons

Communication between brain cells is fundamental to the mechanism by which neurons generate brain function. This communication occurs mainly, but not uniquely, through the release of chemical substances. Chemical communication among nerve cells takes many forms; it may be fast and specific, as it is in synaptic transmission, or it may occur slower and less specifically, as with hormones. In the first instance, specificity means the existence of

a direct contact between given nerve cells. In the case of a hormone, the message is specific only to groups of cells that have receptors for the hormone being released. Although the modes of communication by neurotransmitter and hormones are quite different, it has been found recently that the messenger molecules used in these two modes have much in common. In fact, the same molecule may appear in both types of communication. This is the subject of Chapter 2, "The Molecular Basis of Communication between Cells," by Solomon H. Snyder. While hormones and neurotransmitters have different physiological effects, these messenger molecules are, in other respects, quite similar. This is made clear by Snyder's discussion of the production, release and regulation of sex hormones (estrogens and progesterone). Peptide hormones are also reviewed since some of them (for example, cholesystokinin) also act as neurotransmitters.

This brings us to one of the most exciting discoveries in neuroscience, the class of molecules known as neuropeptides. The enkephalins were chosen by Snyder to exemplify the properties of these molecules. The discovery of neuropeptides demolished two widely held views: one, that transmitters convey only simple "on" (excitation) of "off" (inhibition) messages, and two, that a given presynpatic cell will release a single type of neurotransmitter. (Neuropeptides are also discussed in detail in Chapter 8.)

Neurotransmitters may also bind to second messengers, triggering a cascade of intracellular reactions that have a slow as well as an immediate effect on postsynaptic cells. Second messengers are molecules that trigger biochemical communication between different parts of a cell. The existence of second messengers and the question of how they regulate the biochemistry, cell biology and even the genomic expression of a neuron adds a new and exciting dimension to the study of neuronal function. This topic is covered in Chapter 3, " 'Second Messengers' in the Brain," by James A. Nathanson and Paul Greengard. It demonstrates that nerve cells may be as complex as the circuits in which they are imbedded. The duration of second messenger-mediated events has led the authors to suggest that such events may provide a basis for long-term changes in the nervous system.

As opposed to the slow action of hormones, fast, discrete and specific communication is generally subserved by presynaptic elements releasing neurotransmitter substances that bind to specific receptor molecules on the postsynaptic membrane. In Chapter 4, "Calcium in Synaptic Transmission," I detail the manner in which transmitter is released following the entry of calcium into the presynaptic terminal of the stellate ganglion in the giant squid. A central issue in that chapter is that synaptic transmission is a variation on the theme of secretion and, indirectly, on that of growth. In order for a cell to release transmitter it must fuse internal reservoirs of transmitter substance (membranous microbubbles) with its outer membrane so that the transmitter substance can be secreted. This process is called exocytosis and it is the mechanism by which transmitter and hormones are released to the fluid outside the cell. It is also a mechanism for adding new membrane to the outer cell surface and thus is a form of cell growth.

Among the most important properties of the nervous system is its ability to retain solutions to sensory or motor events that have proven useful in past circumstances. This issue is addressed under the general rubric of memory and learning. Although it is true that these terms entail a complex set of functions probably subserved by many biological mechanisms at many different levels of organization, it is nevertheless essential that we understand the relation of memory and learning to single-cell physiology. The work of Eric Kandel and his colleagues (Chapter 5, "Small Systems of Neurons") illustrates that possible cellular and molecular mechanisms may implement memory in the invertebrate aplysia. This work has led to our understanding of an exciting chapter in neuroscience.

Neurotransmitters

Chapters 6, 7 and 8 concern three quite different aspects of neurotransmitters. Chapter 6, "The Chemical Differentiation of Nerve Cells," by Paul H. Patterson, David D. Potter and Edwin J. Furshpan, is largely concerned with the factors that determine chemical differentiation of neurons in tissue culture, in particular those derived from the autonomic nervous system. These neurons normally differentiate into either cholinergic (acetylcholine releasing) or adrenergic (norepinephrine releasing). The authors discovered that this differentiation is dependent on the composition of the extracellular milieu during a critical period of development. Indeed, a large molecule released from non-neuronal cells (for example, from skeletal or heart muscle cells) can influence the expression of transmitter by these neurons. If these substances are added to cultures lacking non-neuronal elements, cholinergic

cells appear in proportion to the concentration of these molecules added to the media in which the cells grow.

Electrical activity imposed on young cells may also influence whether these cells will be cholinergic or adrenergic: depolarization prevents the induction of cholinergic properties. This is probably mediated by increased intracellular calcium, this ion entering from the extracellular space upon depolarization. These findings bring up the intriguing possibility that the timing and the type of synaptic inputs from the Central Nervous System (CNS) may influence the chemical differentiation of these neurons.

Chapter 7, "GABAergic Neurons," by David I. Gottlieb, considers one group of neurons in detail, those that release the inhibitory neurotransmitters gamma-aminobutyric acid (GABA), one of the important inhibitory transmitters in the CNS. Two types of receptors have been identified for this transmitter substance: $GABA_A$ (activation increases membrane conductance to chloride) and $GABA_B$ (activation increases membrane conductance to potassium). GABAergic cells are found throughout the CNS, comprising the majority of cells in some regions. Gottlieb describes how the amino acid sequence for the receptor was determined. The exciting news is that many chemically sensitive transmembrane channels may be related and be members of a superfamily of molecules that will provide information on exactly how these channels work and how they evolved, probably from a single common ancestor.

Chapter 8, "Neuropeptides," by Floyd E. Bloom, treats that in detail. Two main types of bioactive peptides are used as examples of peptides with long sequences of amino acids. These structures are well conserved in evolution and appear in many species. One type of peptide has short amino acid sequences in common. This group is exemplified by the endorphins and enkephalins. Cells containing the enkephalins are widely distributed in the brain while the endorphins are localized in the region of the hypothalamus and anterior pituitary gland. Genetic engineering tools have been used to determine the amino acid sequence of these neuropeptides. These cells are found in neuronal networks subserving a wide variety of functions. However, cells secreting structurally similar peptides may not be functionally related.

Peptides are special in other respects. They are synthesized only in the ribosomes (in the soma and dendrites, not the axon or axon terminals) as long peptides that are progressively cleaved by specific enzymes into active forms. Their most significant difference from other transmitter molecules is their mode of action. As Bloom puts it, they "disenable" other, traditional transmitters, making them less effective. Each peptide interacts with its own receptor, which must be linked with the receptor for the traditional transmitter. The chapter ends with a discussion of how peptides may mediate behavior.

Nerve Nets

Proceeding from the nature of single cells we next take up the mechanisms by which they communicate with one another. Knowledge of the properties of neuron ensembles, or nerve nets, is vital to understanding brain function. Single cells cannot generate brain properties; such properties are produced by the interactions between nerve cells. This interaction gives rise to the brain as an organ in a manner somewhat analogous to that by which human individuals give rise to politics or economics. Understanding nerve nets is thus a key to understanding the relation between the brain and the mind. Perhaps one of the best-known neuronal networks is in the retina, which covers the inner surface of the eyeball and is responsible for the light sensing that initiates the process of visual perception.

The circuit elements of the retina are more complex than originally thought. It is now known that there are distinct subtypes of the five categories of neurons found in the retina; there may be as many as 50 different functional elements in this network. The properties of the amacrine cell that make only dendrite-to-dendrite connections within the retina (they have no axonic process) are particularly fascinating. Although Ramón y Cajal reported many types of amacrine cells as early as 1892, it was not until recently that many of the neurotransmitters in the brain were also found in these cells, allowing its grouping into different classes.

The question is, how do the rules of connectivity between cells in the retina "encode" the light images into messages. In Chapter 9, "The Functional Architecture of the Retina," Richard H. Masland reviews, on the basis of his own elegant work and that from other laboratories, the possible role of four types of amacrine cells in the retina. He shows that in this neuronal society particular classes of nerve cells are given particular functions, that is, cells "specialize" in the same sense as individuals do. The specializations arise from the particular connectivity (who you know in society) and the types of synaptic interactions (what your contacts tell you and what, in turn, you let your next in line

know about what you have been told). The first to be considered are the acetylcholine-pleasing cells. These excite ganglion cells (the cells that project to the brain). Amacrine cells specialize in "local" signaling. They do not generate action potentials and thus are capable of activating small regions of a dendrite leading to a graded signal with an exquisite spatial localization.

The second type of amacrine cell in the retina is the AII cell. These cells not only sharpen the response of ganglion cells to light but are important for detection of dim light.

The third type of cell was identified by its transmitter, dopamine. These are few of these cells in the retina and their function is still not clear. The last type of amacrine cell discussed by Masland combines the chemical analogues of serotonin and indolamine. These cells come in five "flavors." Because of their synaptic connectivity they are thought to have a major influence on pathways by which dim light passes through the retina, thus providing five different but parallel pathways for the retina to communicate with the brain.

Transplantation

From a medical and a purely experimental vantage point the question of transplanting nerve cells from one brain (or nerve-cell bank) to another is of immense consequence. However, with few exceptions neuronal replacement continues to be only a promise, although it has had great appeal in the neurosciences. Chapter 10, "Transplantation in the Central Nervous System," by Alan Fine, discusses the manner in which cellular events may be modified by implants. The statement has often been made that the nervous system, once having been built, cannot be rebuilt since central nerve cells do not regenerate. This means that, in principal, the genetic heritage for our brain is simultaneously our great provider and our jailer. It implies that whatever we may do to try to correct brain deficits may be achieved only by modifying that which is already present, and probably only in a very subtle and limited manner. But the possibility, however remote, of modifying neuronal networks in a substantial manner—by implanting new neurons—must be carefully studied because it offers the promise that, even in a limited range, we may for the first time be in the position to help brain-injured patients.

Rodolfo R. Llinás

The Biology of the Brain

The Neuron

It is the individual nerve cell, the building block. It transmits nerve impulses over a single long fiber (the axon) and receives them over numerous short fibers (the dendrites).

. . .

Charles F. Stevens

September, 1979

Neurons, or nerve cells, are the building blocks of the brain. Although they have the same genes, the same general organization and the same biochemical apparatus as other cells, they also have unique features that make the brain function in a very different way from, say, the liver. The important specializations of the neuron include a distinctive cell shape, an outer membrane capable of generating nerve impulses, and a unique structure, the synapse, for transferring information from one neuron to the next.

The human brain is thought to consist of 10^{11} neurons, about the same number as the stars in our galaxy. No two neurons are identical in form. Nevertheless, their forms generally fall into only a few broad categories, and most neurons share certain structural features that make it possible to distinguish three regions of the cell: the cell body, the dendrites and the axon. The cell body contains the nucleus of the neuron and the biochemical machinery for synthesizing enzymes and other molecules essential to the life of the cell. Usually the cell body is roughly spherical or pyramid-shaped. The dendrites are delicate tubelike extensions that tend to branch repeatedly and form a bushy tree around the cell body. They provide the main physical surface on which the neuron receives incoming signals. The axon extends away from the cell body and provides the pathway over which signals can travel from the cell body for long distances to other parts of the brain and the nervous system. The axon differs from the dendrites both in structure and in the properties of its outer membrane. Most axons are longer and thinner than dendrites and exhibit a different branching pattern: whereas the branches of dendrites tend to cluster near the cell body, the branches of axons tend to arise at the end of the fiber where the axon communicates with other neurons.

The functioning of the brain depends on the flow of information through elaborate circuits consisting of networks of neurons. Information is transferred from one cell to another at specialized points of contact: the synapses. A typical neuron may have anywhere from 1,000 to 10,000 synapses and may receive information from something like 1,000 other neurons. Although synapses are most often made between the axon of one cell and the dendrite of

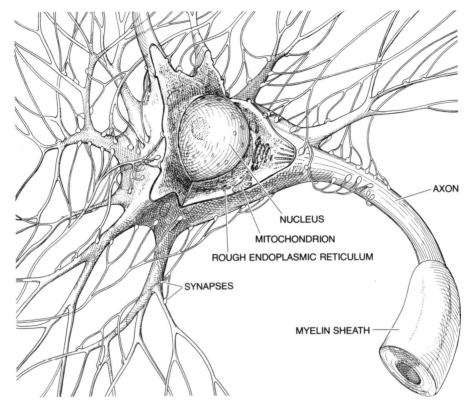

Figure 1 CELL BODY OF A NEURON incorporates the genetic material and complex metabolic apparatus common to all cells, but neurons do not divide after embryonic development; an organism's original supply must serve a lifetime. Projecting from the cell body are several dendrites and a single axon. The cell body and dendrites are covered by synapses. Mitochondria provide the cell with energy. Proteins are synthesized on the endoplasmic reticulum. A transport system moves proteins and other substances from cell body to sites where needed.

another, there are other kinds of synaptic junction: between axon and axon, between dendrite and dendrite and between axon and cell body.

At a synapse the axon usually enlarges to form a terminal button, which is the information-delivering part of the junction. The terminal button contains tiny spherical structures called synaptic vesicles, each of which can hold several thousand molecules of chemical transmitter. On the arrival of a nerve impulse at the terminal button, some of the vesicles discharge their contents into the narrow cleft that separates the button from the membrane of another cell's dendrite, which is designed to receive the chemical message. Hence information is relayed from one neuron to another by means of a transmitter. The "firing" of a neuron—the generation of nerve impulses—reflects the activation of hundreds of synapses by impinging neurons. Some synapses are excitatory in that they tend to promote firing, whereas others are inhibitory and so are capable of canceling signals that otherwise would excite a neuron to fire.

Although neurons are the building blocks of the brain, they are not the only kind of cell in it. For example, oxygen and nutrients are supplied by a dense network of blood vessels. There is also a need for connective tissue, particularly at the surface of the brain. A major class of cells in the central nervous system is the glial cells, or glia. The glia occupy essentially all the space in the nervous system not taken up by the neurons themselves. Although the function of the glia is not fully understood, they provide structural and metabolic support for the delicate meshwork of the neurons.

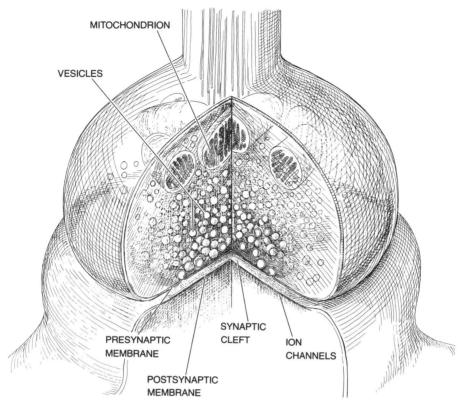

MITOCHONDRION

VESICLES

SYNAPTIC
CLEFT

PRESYNAPTIC
MEMBRANE

ION
CHANNELS

POSTSYNAPTIC
MEMBRANE

Figure 2 SYNAPSE consists of two parts: the knoblike tip of an axon terminal and the receptor region on the surface of another neuron. The membranes are separated by a synaptic cleft some 20 to 30 nanometers across. Molecules of chemical transmitter, stored in vesicles in the axon ter- **minal, are released into the cleft by arriving nerve impulses and change the electrical state of the receiving neuron, making it either more likely or less likely to fire an impulse.**

One other kind of cell, the Schwann cell, is ubiquitous in the nervous system. All axons appear to be jacketed by Schwann cells. In some cases the Schwann cells simply enclose the axon in a thin layer. In many cases, however, the Schwann cell wraps itself around the axon in the course of embryonic development, giving rise to the multiple dense layers of insulation known as myelin. The myelin sheath is interrupted every millimeter or so along the axon by narrow gaps called the nodes of Ranvier. In axons that are sheathed in this way the nerve impulse travels by jumping from node to node, where the extracellular fluid can make direct contact with the cell membrane. The myelin sheath seems to have evolved as a means of conserving the neuron's metabolic energy. In general myelinated nerve fibers conduct nerve impulses faster than unmyelinated fibers.

Neurons can work as they do because their outer membranes have special properties. Along the axon the membrane is specialized to propagate an electrical impulse. At the terminal of the axon the membrane releases transmitters, and on the dendrites it responds to transmitters. In addition the membrane mediates the recognition of other cells in embryonic development, so that each cell finds its proper place in the network of 10^{11} cells. Much recent investigation therefore focuses on the membrane properties responsible for the nerve impulse, for synaptic transmission, for cell-cell recognition and for structural contacts between cells.

The neuron membrane, like the outer membrane of all cells, is about five nanometers thick and consists of two layers of lipid molecules arranged with their hydrophilic ends pointing toward the water on the inside and outside of the cell and with their

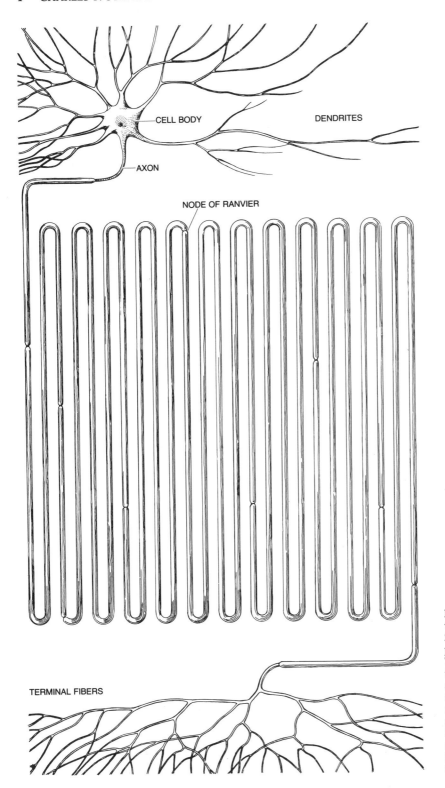

CELL BODY

DENDRITES

AXON

NODE OF RANVIER

TERMINAL FIBERS

Figure 3 TYPICAL NEURON of a vertebrate animal (enlarged here 225 times) can carry nerve impulses for a considerable distance. The nerve impulses originate in the cell body and are propagated along the axon. This axon, folded for the diagram, would be a centimeter long at actual size, although some axons are more than a meter long. Many axons are insulated by a myelin sheath interrupted at intervals by the regions known as nodes of Ranvier.

hydrophobic ends pointing away from the water to form the interior of the membrane. The lipid parts of the membrane are about the same for all kinds of cells. What makes one cell membrane different from another are various specific proteins that are associated with the membrane in one way or another. Proteins that are actually embedded in the lipid bilayer are termed intrinsic proteins. Other proteins, the peripheral membrane proteins, are attached to the membrane surface but do not form an integral part of its structure. Because the membrane lipid is fluid even the intrinsic proteins are often free to move by diffusion from place to place. In some instances, however, the proteins are firmly fastened down by a substructure.

The membrane proteins of all cells fall into five classes: pumps, channels, receptors, enzymes and structural proteins. Pumps expend metabolic energy to move ions and other molecules against concentration gradients in order to maintain appropriate concentrations of these molecules within the cell. Because charged molecules do not pass through the lipid bilayer itself cells have evolved channel proteins that provide selective pathways through which specific ions can diffuse. Cell membranes must recognize and attach many types of molecules. Receptor proteins fulfill these functions by providing binding sites with great specificity and high affinity. Enzymes are placed in or on the membrane to facilitate chemical reactions at the membrane surface. Finally, structural proteins both interconnect cells to form organs and help to maintain subcellular structure. These five classes of membrane proteins are not necessarily mutually exclusive. For example, a particular protein might simultaneously be a receptor, an enzyme and a pump.

Membrane proteins are the key to understanding neuron function and therefore brain function. Because they play such a central role in modern views of the neuron, I shall organize my discussion around a description of an ion pump, various types of channel and some other proteins that taken together endow neurons with their unique properties. The general idea will be to summarize the important characteristics of the membrane proteins and to explain how these characteristics account for the nerve impulse and other complex features of neuron function.

Like all cells the neuron is able to maintain within itself a fluid whose composition differs markedly from that of the fluid outside it. The difference is particularly striking with regard to the concentration of the ions of sodium and potassium. The external medium is about 10 times richer in sodium than the internal one, and the internal medium is about 10 times richer in potassium than the external one. Both sodium and potassium leak through pores in the cell membrane, so that a pump must operate continuously to exchange sodium ions that have entered the cell for potassium ions outside it. The pumping is accomplished by an intrinsic membrane protein called the sodium-potassium adenosine triphosphatase pump, or more often simply the sodium pump.

The protein molecule (or complex of protein subunits) of the sodium pump has a molecular weight of about 275,000 daltons and measures roughly six by eight nanometers, or slightly more than the thickness of the cell membrane. Each sodium pump can harness the energy stored in the phosphate bond of adenosine triphosphate (ATP) to exchange three sodium ions on the inside of the cell for two potassium ions on the outside. Operating at the maximum rate, each pump can transport across the membrane some 200 sodium ions and 130 potassium ions per second. The actual rate, however, is adjusted to meet the needs of the cell. Most neurons have between 100 and 200 sodium pumps per square micrometer of membrane surface, but in some parts of their surface the density is as much as 10 times higher. A typical small neuron has perhaps a million sodium pumps with a capacity to move about 200 million sodium ions per second. It is the transmembrane gradients of sodium and potassium ions that enable the neuron to propagate nerve impulses.

Membrane proteins that serve as channels are essential for many aspects of neuron function, particularly for the nerve impulse and synaptic transmission. As an introduction to the role played by channels in the electrical activity of the brain, I shall briefly describe the mechanism of the nerve impulse and then return to a more systematic survey of channel properties.

Since the concentration of sodium and potassium ions on one side of the cell membrane differs from that on the other side, the interior of the axon is about 70 millivolts negative with respect to the exterior. In their classic studies of nerve-impulse transmission in the giant axon of the squid a quarter of a century ago, A. L. Hodgkin, A. F. Huxley and Bernhard Katz of Britain demonstrated that the propagation of the nerve impulse coincides with sudden

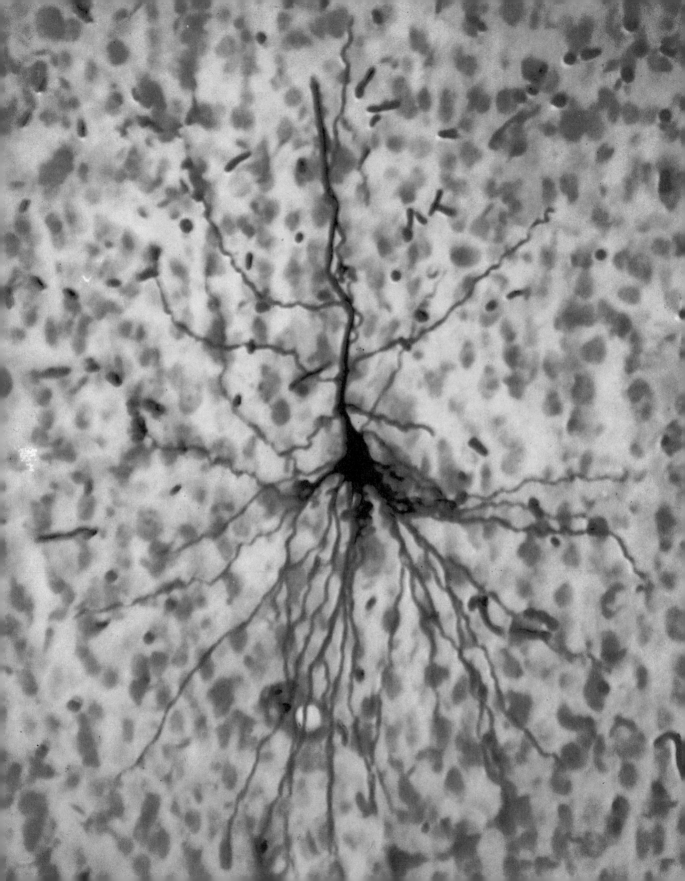

Figure 4 NEURON FROM A CAT'S VISUAL CORTEX labeled in a micrograph by injection with horseradish peroxidase. The wavy processes extending from the cell body are dendrites. The axon is much finer and not readily visible at this magnification. The thickest processes, extending vertically upward, is the apical dendrite. The activity of this cell was recorded in the living animal and was found to respond optimally to a light-dark border rotated about 60 degrees from the vertical. (Micrograph by C. Gilbert and T. N. Wiesel of Harvard Medical School.)

changes in the permeability of the axon membrane to sodium and potassium ions. When a nerve impulse starts at the origin of the axon, having been triggered in most cases by the cell body in response to dendritic synapses, the voltage difference across the axon membrane is locally lowered. Immediately ahead of the electrically altered region (in the direction in which the nerve impulse is propagated) channels in the membrane open and let sodium ions pour into the axon.

The process is self-reinforcing: the flow of sodium ions through the membrane opens more channels and makes it easier for other ions to follow. The sodium ions that enter change the internal potential of the membrane from negative to positive. Soon after the sodium channels open they close, and another group of channels open that let potassium ions flow out. This outflow restores the voltage inside the axon to its resting value of −70 millivolts. The sharp positive and then negative charge, which shows up as a "spike" on an oscilloscope, is known as the action potential and is the electrical manifestation of the nerve impulse. The wave of voltage

sweeps along until it reaches the end of the axon much as a flame travels along the fuse of a firecracker.

This brief description of the nerve impulse illustrates the importance of channels for the electrical activity of neurons and underscores two fundamental properties of channels: selectivity and gating. I shall discuss these two properties in turn. Channels are selectively permeable and selectivities vary widely. For example, one type of channel lets sodium ions pass through and largely excludes potassium ions, whereas another type of channel does the reverse. The selectivity, however, is seldom absolute. One type of channel that is fairly nonselective allows the passage of about 85 sodium ions for every 100 potassium ions; another more selective type passes only about seven sodium ions for every 100 potassium ions. The first type, known as the acetylcholine-activated channel, has a pore about .8 nanometer in diameter that is filled with water. The second type, known as the potassium channel, has a much smaller opening and contains less water.

The sodium ion is about 30 percent smaller than the potassium ion. The exact molecular structure that enables the larger ion to pass through the cell membrane more readily than the smaller one is not known. The general principles that underlie the discrimination, however, are understood. They involve interactions between ions and parts of the channel structure in conjunction with a particular ordering of water molecules within the pore.

The gating mechanism that regulates the opening and closing of membrane channels takes two main

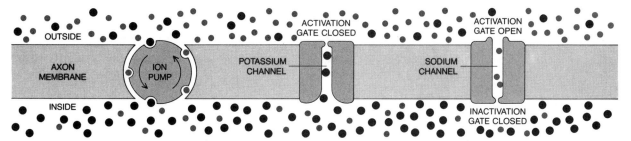

Figure 5 AXON MEMBRANE separates fluids that differ greatly in their content (a disequilibrium). Sodium ions (*colored dots*) are high outside and potassium ions (*black dots*) are high inside. The membrane is penetrated by proteins that act as selective ionic channels. In the resting state, when no nerve impulse is transmitted, the sodium and potassium channels are closed and an ion pump maintains the ionic disequilibrium. If voltage across the membrane is reduced, the sodium channels open and sodium ions enter the axon. An instant later the sodium channels close and the potassium channels open and potassium ions exit the axon. This sequence of events generates the nerve impulse.

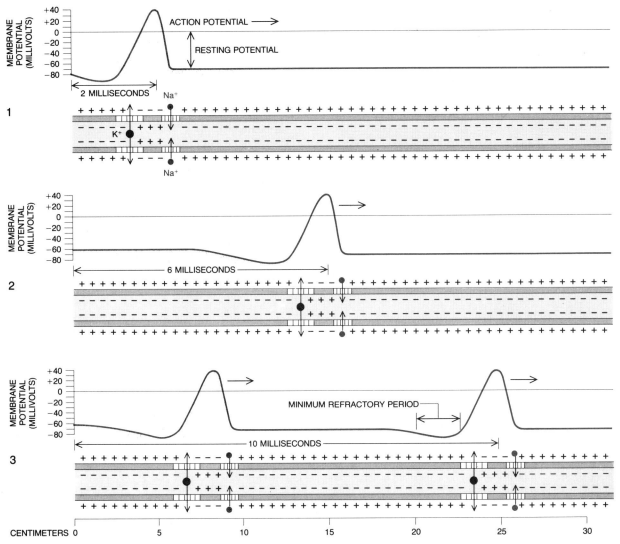

Figure 6 NERVE IMPULSE, as measured in the giant axon of the squid, begins with a slight reduction in the negative potential across the membrane of the axon at its junction with the cell body, which opens some sodium channels, shifting the voltage further. The inflow of sodium ions (Na^+) accelerates until the inner surface of the membrane is locally positive. The voltage reversal closes the sodium channel and opens the potassium channel. The outflow of potassium ions (K^+) quickly restores the negative potential. This voltage reversal, or action potential, propagates itself down the axon (1, 2). After a brief refractory period a second impulse can follow (3).

forms. One type of channel, mentioned above in the description of the nerve impulse, opens and closes in response to voltage differences across the cell membrane; it is therefore said to be voltage-gated. A second type of channel is chemically gated. Such channels respond only slightly if at all to voltage changes but open when a particular molecule—a transmitter—binds to a receptor region on the channel protein. Chemically gated channels are found in the receptive membranes of synapses and are responsible for translating the chemical signals produced by axon terminals into ion permeability changes during synaptic transmission. It is customary to name chemically gated channels according to their normal transmitter. Hence one speaks of acetylcholine-activated channels or GABA-activated channel (GABA is a gamma-aminobutyric acid.) Voltage-gated channels are generally named for the ion that passes through the channel most readily.

Proteins commonly change their shape as they function. Such alterations in shape, known as conformational changes, are dramatic for the contractile proteins responsible for cell motion, but they are no less important in many enzymes and other proteins. Conformational changes in channel proteins form the basis for gating as they serve to open and close the channel by slight movements of critically placed portions of the molecule that unblock and block the pore.

When either voltage-gated or chemically gated channels open and allow ions to pass, one can measure the resulting electric current. Quite recently it has become possible in a few instances to record the current flowing through a single channel, so that the opening and closing can be directly detected. One finds that the length of time a channel stays open varies randomly because the opening and closing of the channel represents a change in the conformation of the protein molecule embedded in the membrane. The random nature of the gating process arises from the haphazard collision of water molecules and other molecules with the structural elements of the channel.

In addition to ion pumps and channels, neurons depend on other classes of membrane proteins for carrying out essential nervous-system functions. One of the important proteins is the enzyme adenylate cyclase, which helps to regulate the intracellular substance cyclic adenosine monophosphate (cyclic AMP). Cyclic nucleotides such as cyclic AMP take part in cell functions whose mechanisms are not yet understood in detail. The membrane enzyme adenylate cyclase appears to have two chief subunits, one catalytic and the other regulatory. The catalytic subunit promotes the formation of cyclic AMP. Various regulatory subunits, which are thought to be physically distinct from the catalytic one, can bind specific molecules (including transmitters that open and close channels) in order to control intracellular levels of cyclic AMP. The various types of regulatory subunit are named according to the molecule that normally binds to them; one, for example, is called serotonin-activated adenylate cyclase. Adenylate cyclase and related membrane enzymes are known to serve a number of regulatory functions in

neurons, and the precise mechanisms of these actions are now under active investigation.

In the course of the embryonic development of the nervous system a cell must be able to recognize other cells so that the growth of each cell will proceed in the right direction and give rise to the right connections. The process of cell-cell recognition and the maintenance of the structure arrived at by such recognition depend on special classes of membrane proteins that are associated with unusual carbohydrates. The study of the protein-carbohydrate complexes associated with cell recognition is still at an early stage.

The intrinsic membrane proteins I have been describing are neither distributed uniformly over the cell surface nor all present in equal amounts in each neuron. The density and the type of protein are governed by the needs of the cell and differ among types of neuron and from one region of a neuron to another. Thus the density of channels of a particular type ranges from zero up to about 10,000 per square micrometer. Axons generally have no chemically gated channels, whereas in postsynaptic membranes the density of such channels is limited only by the packing of the channel molecules. Similarly, dendritic membranes typically have few voltage-gated channels, whereas in axon membranes the density can reach 1,000 channels per square micrometer in certain locations.

The intrinsic membrane proteins are synthesized primarily in the body of the neuron and are stored in the membrane in small vesicles. Neurons have a special transport system for moving such vesicles from their site of synthesis to their site of function. The transport system seems to move the vesicles along in small jumps with the aid of contractile proteins. On reaching their destination the proteins are inserted into the surface membrane, where they function until they are removed and degraded within the cell. Precisely how the cell decides where to put which membrane protein is not known. Equally unknown is the mechanism that regulates the synthesis, insertion and destruction of the membrane proteins. The metabolism of membrane proteins constitutes one of cell biology's central problems.

How do the properties of the various membrane proteins I have been discussing relate to neuron function? To approach this question let us now return to the nerve impulse and examine more closely the molecular properties that underlie its triggering

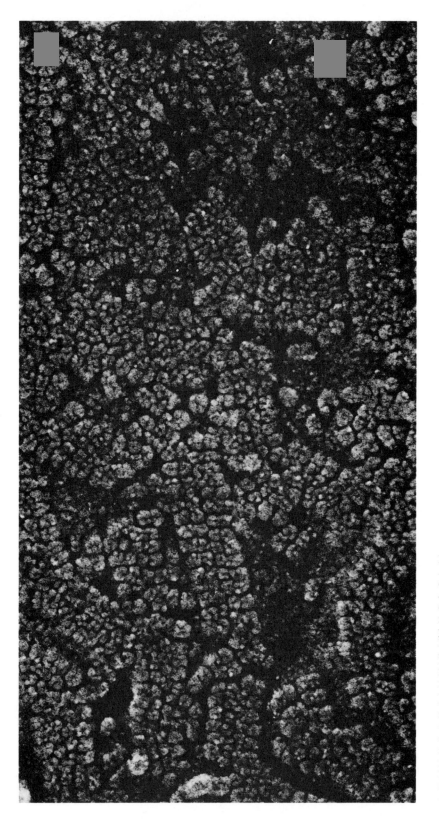

Figure 7 ACETYLCHOLINE-ACTIVATED CHANNELS are densely packed in the postsynaptic membrane of a cell in the electric organ of a torpedo. This micrograph shows the platinum-plated replica of a membrane that had been frozen and etched. The size of the platinum particles limits the resolution to features larger than about two nanometers. Recent evidence shows that the channel protein molecule, which measures 8.5 nanometers across, consists of five subunits surrounding a channel whose narrowest dimension is 0.8 nanometer. (Micrograph by J. E. Heuser, University of California School of Medicine in San Francisco, and S. R. Saltpeter.)

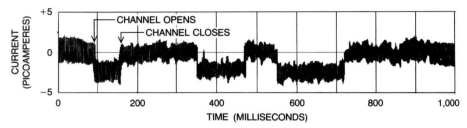

Figure 8 RESPONSE OF A SINGLE MEMBRANE CHAN-NEL to acetylcholine. Acetylcholine-activated channels allow the passage of roughly equal numbers of sodium and potassium ions. The record shows the flow of current through a single channel in the postsynaptic membrane of a frog muscle activated by suberyldicholine, which mimics acetylcholine but keeps channels open longer. Experiment shows that channels open on an all-or-none basis and stay open for random lengths of time.

and propagation. As we have seen, the interior of the neuron is about 70 millivolts negative with respect to the exterior. This "resting potential" is a consequence of the ionic disequilibrium brought about by the sodium pump and by the presence in the cell membrane of a class of permanently open channels selectively permeable to potassium ions. The pump ejects sodium ions, in exchange for potassium ions, making the inside of the cell about 10 times richer in potassium ions than the outside. The potassium channels in the membrane allow the potassium ions immediately adjacent to the membrane to flow outward quite freely. The permeability of the membrane to sodium ions is low in the resting condition, so that there is almost no counterflow of sodium ions from the exterior to the interior even though the external medium is tenfold richer in sodium ions than the internal medium. The potassium flow therefore gives rise to a net deficit of positive charges on the inner surface of the cell membrane and an excess of positive charges on the outer surface. The result is the voltage difference of 70 millivolts, with the interior being negative.

The propagation of the nerve impulse depends on the presence in the neuron membrane of voltage-gated sodium channels whose opening and closing is responsible for the action potential. What are the characteristics of these important channel molecules? Although the sodium channel has not yet been well characterized chemically, it is a protein with a molecular weight probably in the range of 250,000 to 300,000 daltons. The pore of the channel measures about .4 by .6 nanometer, a space through which sodium ions can pass in association with a water molecule. The channel has many charged groups critically placed on its surface. These charges

give the channel a large electric dipole moment that varies in direction and magnitude when the molecular conformation of the channel changes as the channel goes from a closed state to an open one.

Because the surface membrane of the cell is so thin the difference of 70 millivolts across the resting membrane gives rise to a large electric field, on the order of 100 kilovolts per centimeter. In the same way that magnetic dipoles tend to align themselves with the lines of force in a magnetic field, the electric dipoles in the sodium-channel protein tend to align themselves with the membrane electric field. Changes in the strength of the membrane field can therefore drive the channel from the closed conformation to the open one. As the inner surface of the membrane is made more positive by the entering vanguard of sodium ions, the sodium channels tend to spend an increasing fraction of their time in the open conformation. The process in which the channels are opened by a change in the membrane voltage is known as sodium-channel activation.

The process is terminated by a phenomenon called sodium inactivation. Voltage differences across the membrane that cause sodium channels to open also drive them into a special closed conformation different from the conformation characteristic of the channel's resting state. The second closed conformation, called the inactivated state, develops more slowly than the activation process, so that channels remain open briefly before they are closed by inactivation. The channels remain in the inactivated state for some milliseconds and then return to the normal resting state.

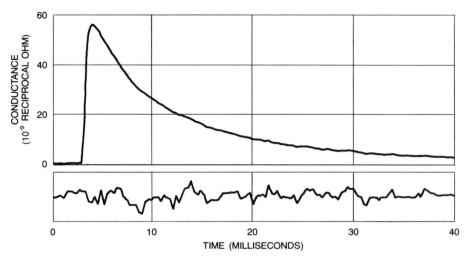

Figure 9 SODIUM CHANNELS IN AN AXON operate in simple open-or-shut manner and independently of one another. During propagation of a nerve impulse about 10,000 channels open in a node of Ranvier. The upper trace depicts the sodium permeability at such a node as a function of time. The lower trace, recorded at a 12-fold amplification of the upper one, shows fluctuations in permeability around the average due to random opening and closing of channels.

The complete cycle of activation and inactivation normally involves the opening and closing of thousands of sodium channels. How can one tell whether the increase in overall membrane permeability reflects the opening and closing of a number of channels in an all-or-none manner or whether it reflects the operation of channels that have individually graded permeabilities? The question has been partly answered by a new technique that relates fluctuations in membrane permeability to the inherently probabilistic nature of conformational changes in the channel proteins. One can trigger repeated

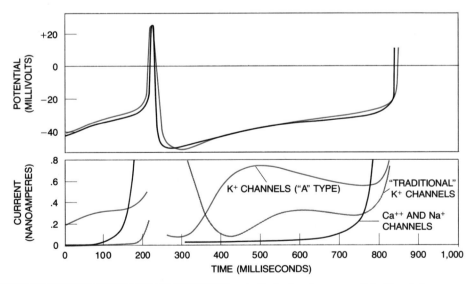

Figure 10 NERVE IMPULSES IN BODIES OF NEURONS require the coordinated opening and closing of five types of channel permeable to various kinds of ion (sodium, potassium or calcium). The upper pair of curves represent an actual recording of voltage changes as a function of time in the body of a neuron (*black*) and changes computed from equations (*color*). The lower curves depict the current carried by the principal types of channel as a function of time. A complicated interaction of channel types is required to achieve a train of nerve impulses.

episodes of channel opening and calculate the average permeability at a particular time and also the exact permeability on a given trial. The exact permeability fluctuates 10 percent or so around a mean value. Analysis of the fluctuations shows that the sodium channels open in an all-or-none manner and that each channel opening increases the conductance of the membrane by 8×10^{-12} reciprocal ohms. One of the principal challenges in understanding the neuron is the development of a complete theory that will describe the behavior of the sodium channels and relate it to the molecular structure of the channel protein.

As I noted briefly above, axons also have voltage-gated potassium channels that help to terminate the nerve impulse by letting potassium ions flow out of the axon, thereby counteracting the inward flow of sodium ions. In the cell body of the neuron the situation is still more complex, because there the membrane is traversed by five types of channel. The different channels open at different rates, stay open for various intervals and are preferentially permeable to different species of ions (sodium, potassium or calcium).

The presence of the five types of channel in the cell body of the neuron, compared with only two in the axon, gives rise to a more complex mode of nerve-impulse generation. If an axon is presented with a maintained stimulus, it generates only a single impulse at the onset of the stimulus. Cell bodies, however, generate a train of impulses with a frequency that reflects the intensity of the stimulus.

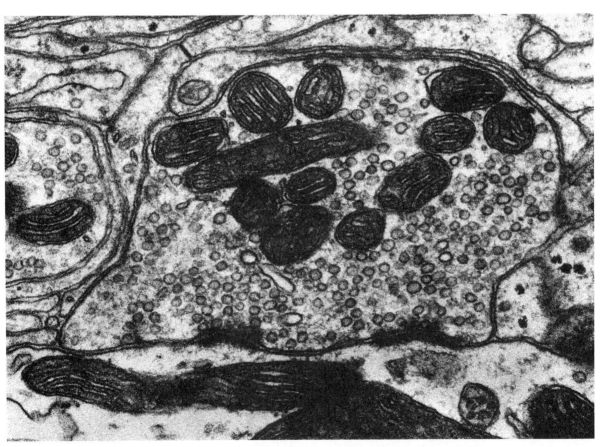

Figure 11 SYNAPTIC TERMINAL. The cleft separating the presynaptic membrane from the postsynaptic one undulates across the lower part of the micrograph. The large dark structures are mitochondria. The many round bodies are vesicles that hold transmitter. The fuzzy dark thickenings along the cleft are thought to be principal sites of transmitter release. (Micrograph by J. E. Heuser, and T. S. Reese of the National Institutes of Health.)

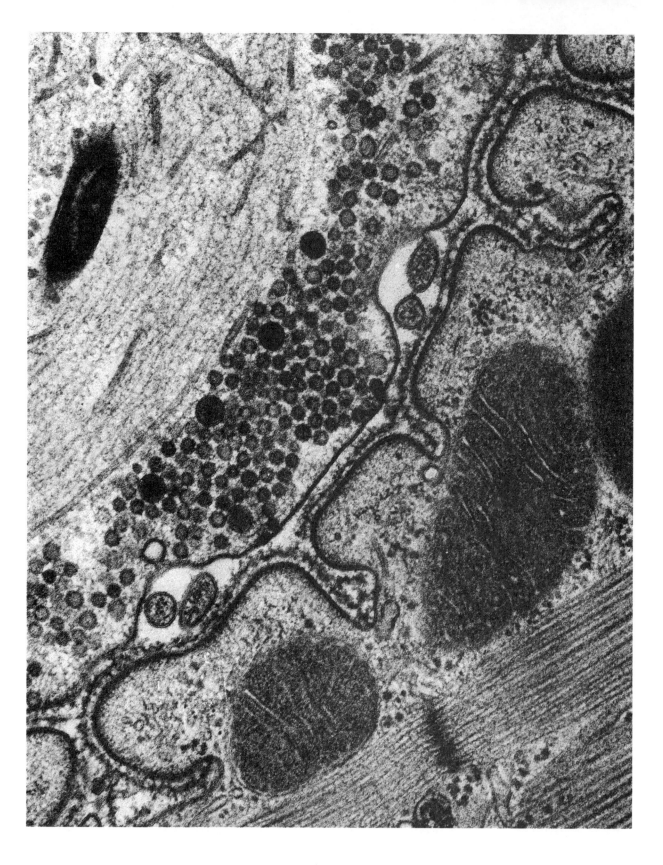

Figure 12 FROG NEUROMUSCULAR JUNCTION. The synaptic cleft separates the axon at the upper left from the muscle cell at the lower right. Synaptic vesicles cluster along the presynaptic membrane, with two synaptic contacts visible near the center. Postsynaptic membrane of the muscle cell exhibits a feature that is not seen at other synapses: the membrane forms postjunctional folds opposite each contact. (Micrograph by J. E. Heuser.)

Neurons are able to generate nerve impulses over a wide range of frequencies, from one or fewer per second to several hundred per second. All nerve impulses have the same amplitude, so that the information they carry is represented by the number of impulses generated per unit of time, a system known as frequency coding. The larger the magnitude of the stimulus to be conveyed, the faster the rate of firing.

When a nerve impulse has traveled the length of the axon and has arrived at a terminal button, one of a variety of transmitters is released from the presynaptic membrane. The transmitter diffuses to the postsynaptic membrane, where it induces the opening of chemically gated channels. Ions flowing through the open channels bring about the voltage changes known as postsynaptic potentials.

Most of what is known about synaptic mechanisms comes from experiments on a particular synapse: the neuromuscular junction that controls the contraction of muscles in the frog. The axon of the frog neuron runs for several hundred micrometers along the surface of the muscle cell, making several hundred synaptic contacts spaced about a micrometer apart. At each presynaptic region the characteristic synaptic vesicles can be recognized readily.

Each of the synaptic vesicles contains some 10,000 molecules of the transmitter acetylcholine. When a nerve impulse reaches the synapse, a train of events is set in motion that culminates in the fusion of a vesicle with the presynaptic membrane and the resulting release of acetylcholine into the cleft between the presynaptic and the postsynaptic membranes, a process termed exocytosis. The fused vesicle is subsequently reclaimed from the presynaptic membrane and is quickly refilled with acetylcholine for future release.

Many details of the events leading to exocytosis have recently been elucidated. The fusion of vesicles to the presynaptic membrane is evidently triggered by a rapid but transient increase in the concentration of calcium in the terminal button of the axon. The arrival of a nerve impulse at the terminal opens calcium channels that are voltage-gated and allows calcium to flow into the terminal. The subsequent rise in calcium concentration is brief, however, because the terminal contains a special apparatus that rapidly sequesters free calcium and returns its concentration to the normal very low

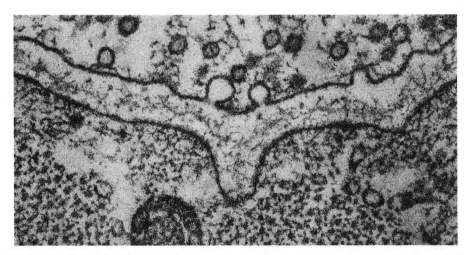

Figure 13 TRANSMITTER IS DISCHARGED into the synaptic cleft at the synaptic junctions between neurons by vesicles that open up after they fuse with the axon's presynaptic membrane, a process called exocytosis. This micrograph has caught the vesicles in the terminal of an axon in the act of discharging acetylcholine into the neuromuscular junction of a frog. The structures in the micrograph are enlarged 115,000 diameters. (Micrograph by J. E. Heuser.)

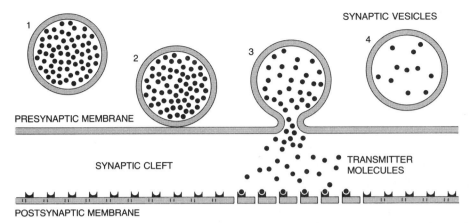

Figure 14 SYNAPTIC VESICLES are clustered near the presynaptic membrane. The diagram shows the probable steps in exocytosis. Filled vesicles move up to synaptic cleft, fuse with the membrane, discharge their contents and are reclaimed, re-formed and refilled with transmitter.

level. The brief spike in the free-calcium level leads to the fusion of transmitter-filled vesicles with the presynaptic membrane, but the precise mechanism of this important process is not yet known.

Interesting details of the structure of the terminal membrane have been revealed by the freeze-fracture technique, a method that splits the layers of the bilayer membrane and exposes the intrinsic membrane proteins for examination by electron microscopy. In the frog neuromuscular junction a double row of large membrane proteins runs the width of each synapse. Synaptic vesicles become attached on or near the proteins. Only these vesicles then fuse to the membrane and release their transmitter; other vesicles seem to be held in reserve some distance away. The fusion of vesicles is a random process and occurs independently for each vesicle.

In less than 100 microseconds acetylcholine released from fused vesicles diffuses across the synaptic cleft and binds to the acetylcholine receptor: an intrinsic membrane protein embedded in the postsynaptic membrane. The receptor is also a channel protein that is chemically gated by the presence of acetylcholine. When two acetylcholine molecules attach themselves to the channel, they lower the energy state of the open conformation of the protein and thereby increase the probability that the channel will open. The open state of the channel is a random event with an average lifetime of about a millisecond. Each packet of 10,000 acetylcholine molecules effects the opening of some 2,000 channels.

During the brief period that a channel is open about 20,000 sodium ions and a roughly equal number of potassium ions pass through it. As a result of this ionic flow the voltage difference between the two sides of the membrane tends to approach zero. How close it approaches to zero depends on how many channels open and how long they stay open. The acetylcholine released by a typical nerve impulse produces a postsynaptic potential, or voltage change, that lasts for only about five milliseconds. Because postsynaptic potentials are produced by chemically gated channels rather than by voltage-gated ones, they have properties quite different from those of the nerve impulse. They are usually smaller in amplitude, longer in duration and graded in size depending on the quantity of transmitter released and hence on the number of channels that open.

Different types of chemically gated channels exhibit different selectivities. Some resemble the acetylcholine channel, which passes sodium and potassium ions with little selectivity. Others are highly selective. The voltage change that results at a particular synapse depends on the selectivity of the channels that are opened. If positive ions move into the cell, the voltage change is in the positive direction. Such positive-going voltage channels tend to open voltage-gated channels and to generate nerve impulses, and so they are known as excitatory postsynaptic potentials. If positive ions (usually potassium) move out of the cell, the voltage change is in the negative direction, which tends to close voltage-gated channels. Such postsynaptic potentials oppose the production of nerve impulses, and so they are termed inhibitory. Excitatory and inhibitory postsynaptic potentials are both common in the brain.

Brain synapses differ from neuromuscular-junction synapses in several ways. Whereas at the neuromuscular junction the action of acetylcholine is always excitatory, in the brain the action of the same substance is excitatory at some synapses and inhibitory at others. And whereas acetylcholine is the usual transmitter at neuromuscular junctions, the brain synapses have channels gated by a large variety of transmitters. A particular synaptic ending, however, releases only one type of transmitter, and channels gated by that transmitter are present in the corresponding postsynaptic membrane. In contrast with neuromuscular channels activated by acetylcholine, which stay open for about a millisecond, some types of brain synapses have channels that remain open for hundreds of milliseconds. A final major difference is that whereas the axon makes hundreds of synaptic contacts with the muscle cell at the frog's neuromuscular junction, axons in the brain usually make only one or two synaptic contacts on a given neuron. As might be expected, such different functional properties are correlated with significant differences in structure.

As we have seen, the intensity of a stimulus is coded in the frequency of nerve impulses. Decoding at the synapse is accomplished by two processes: temporal summation and spatial summation.

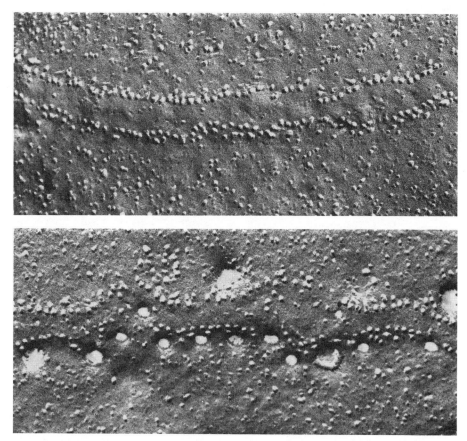

Figure 15 FREEZE-FRACTURE REPLICAS of the presynaptic membrane of the frog neuromuscular junction. The upper micrograph shows the membrane three milliseconds after the muscle had been stimulated. Running across the axon membrane is a double row of membrane proteins that may be calcium channels or structural proteins to which vesicles attach. The lower micrograph shows the membrane five milliseconds after stimulation, which has caused synaptic vesicles to fuse with presynaptic membrane and form pits. (Micrographs by J. E. Heuser.)

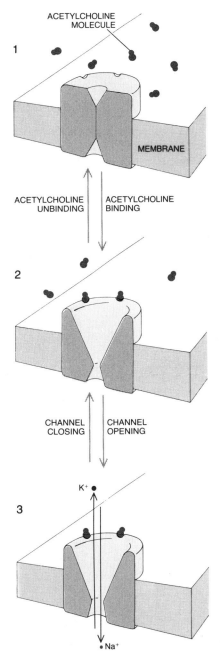

1

ACETYLCHOLINE
MOLECULE

MEMBRANE

ACETYLCHOLINE
UNBINDING

ACETYLCHOLINE
BINDING

2

CHANNEL
CLOSING

CHANNEL
OPENING

K+ •

3

• Na+

Figure 16 ACETYLCHOLINE CHANNEL in a postsynaptic membrane is opened by acetylcholine molecules discharging into the synaptic cleft. Two molecules bind rapidly to the resting closed channel to form a receptor-acetylcholine complex (1, 2), which undergoes a conformation change that opens the channel to about 20,000 sodium and 20,000 potassium ions (3). The time required for conformational change limits the speed of the reaction. The channel remains open for about a millisecond and reverts to the receptor-acetylcholine complex. The acetylcholine rapidly dissociates and is destroyed by the enzyme acetylcholine esterase.

In temporal summation each postsynaptic potential adds to the cumulative total of its predecessors to yield a voltage change whose average amplitude reflects the frequency of incoming nerve impulses. In other words, a neuron that is firing rapidly releases more transmitter molecules at its terminal junctions than a neuron that is firing less rapidly. The more transmitter molecules that are released in a given time, the more channels that are opened in the postsynaptic membrane and therefore the larger the postsynaptic potential is. Spatial summation is an equivalent process except that it reflects the integration of nerve impulses arriving from all the neurons that may be in synaptic contact with a given neuron. The grand voltage change derived by temporal and spatial summation is encoded as nerve-impulse frequency for transmission to other cells "downstream" in the nerve network.

I have described what is usually regarded as the normal flow of information in neural circuits, in which postsynaptic voltage changes are encoded as nerve-impulse frequency and transmitted over the axon to other neurons. In recent years, however, a number of instances have been discovered where a postsynaptic potential is not converted into a nerve impulse. For example, the voltage change due to a postsynaptic potential can directly cause the release of transmitter from a neighboring site that lacks a nerve impulse. Such direct influences are thought to come into play in synapses between dendrites and also in certain reciprocal circuits where one dendrite makes a synaptic contact on a second dendrite, which in turn makes a synaptic contact back on the first dendrite. Such direct feedback seems to be quite common in the brain, but its implications for information processing remain to be worked out.

Much current investigation of the neuron focuses on the membrane proteins that endow the cell's bilayer membrane, which is otherwise featureless, with the special properties brain function depends on. With regard to channel proteins there are many unanswered questions about the mechanisms of gating, selectivity and regulation. Within the next five or 10 years it should be possible to relate the physical processes of gating and selectivity to the molecular structure of the channels. The basis of channel regulation is less well understood but is now coming under intensive investigation. It seems that hormones and other substances play a role in channel regulation that is now becoming appreciated. The central problems at synaptic junctions involve exocytosis and other activities related to the metabolism and release of transmitters. One can expect increasing attention to be focused on the role of the surface membrane in the growth and development of neurons and their synaptic connections, the remarkable process that establishes the integration of the nervous system.

POSTSCRIPT

The issue of how the electrical activity of central neurons (neurons in the brain) relates to their ability to transfer information is currently one of the most exciting areas in neuroscience. While in the past such cells were assumed to be little more than relays, as we unravel the molecular and biophysical nature of neuronal activity we understand that neurons are "brighter" than we ever imagined. They are in fact endowed with an incredibly rich set of mechanisms for the expression of messages, to the point of message creativity as it happens in dreams. Three general categories of ion channels are recognized at the molecular level and their amino acid structure has been sequenced. The first category is the voltage-sensitive channels that demonstrate different degrees of selectivity for sodium, potassium and calcium ions. The second category is the channels activated by chemical transmitter substances, such as the nicotinic ACh channel, the acidic amino acid transmitter (glutamic and aspartic acid channels) and the inhibitory channel activated by GABA or glycine that allows chloride through. The molecular structure of the first two categories of channels suggests that they may belong to the same superfamily. The third category is the chemically activated channels that require an intermediate biochemical step. Thus the receptor is coupled through a moiety known as a G protein to a cyclase; G proteins can have an inhibitory or excitatory effect on the ionic conductances they regulate. Examples are the muscarinic ACh receptors, dopamine receptors and the rhodopsin molecules in the photoreceptors of the eye (see works by Numa, 1986 and Kosower, 1988). Because all three categories of channels are now recognized in central neurons, their role in neuronal integration is presently being explored.

In addition, some of the ligand-gated receptors have recently been shown to be modulated by membrane voltage; in particular, the N-methyl D aspartate (NMDA) receptor in central neurons responds poorly to the transmitter glutamic acid at the resting potentials, but increases its responsiveness quite dramatically if the membrane is depolarized (made less negative). This happens because Mg^{++}, which is normally logged in the channel aqueous pore of the channel, pops out when the membrane potential changes, allowing more ions to flow when the channels are activated by glutamic acid. This phenomenon has been related to some aspects of synaptic potentiations that may be related to memory acquisition (see review by Cotman and Iversen, 1988).

From a more integrative point of view, the electrophysiology of the nervous system has gained from the in vitro slice studies and isolated single cells in the past decade, using intracellular recording or patch-clamp techniques (Francioline and Petris, 1988; Neher, 1988). Results from such studies indicate that many more different types of voltage- and chemically-gated channels are present in central neurons than previously suspected. The results indicate that, in addition to synaptic mediated activity, central neurons can have spontaneous, oscillatory activity produced by the interplay of the different voltage-dependent channels within the membrane of a single cell (Llinás, 1989).

The Molecular Basis of Communication between Cells

Chemical messengers mediate long-range hormonal communication and short-range communication between nerve cells. The two systems differ in directness, but some messenger molecules are common to both.

• • •

Solomon H. Snyder

October, 1985

The unicellular amoeba can perform every function necessary to sustain life. The cell can assimilate nutrients from the environment, move itself about and carry out the metabolic reactions that provide it with energy and synthesize new cellular molecules. In multicellular organisms the situation is considerably more complex. The various tasks are split up among many distinct cell populations, tissues and organs, which may be far apart from one another. To coordinate all these various functions there must be mechanisms whereby individual cells or groups of cells can communicate with one another.

In most higher organisms there are two primary methods of communication between cells: systems of hormones and systems of neurons, or nerve cells. In both systems cells "talk" to one another by means of chemical messengers. The main difference between the two systems is the level of directness with which they act. A neuron sends discrete messages to a specific set of target cells: muscle cells, gland cells or other neurons. To send a message the neuron releases a chemical called a neurotransmit-

ter toward the target cell. The cell-to-cell communication takes place at specific sites known as synapses. Molecules of neurotransmitter become attached to receptors (usually protein molecules) on the surface of the target cell and effect chemical changes at the cell membrane and within the cell itself.

Hormone action is usually less direct. Although so-called autocrine and paracrine mechanisms exist, in which a hormone acts respectively on the cell that released it or on an adjacent cell, the commonest form of hormonal communication is in the endocrine system, where a gland releases hormones that may act on cells or organs anywhere in the body. Endocrine glands secrete hormones into the bloodstream; each target cell is equipped with receptors that recognize only the hormone molecules meant to act on that cell. The receptors pull the hormone molecules out of the bloodstream and bring them into the cell.

There are thus considerable differences between hormonal and neural communication. Neurons tend to act over short distances on a particular cell or set

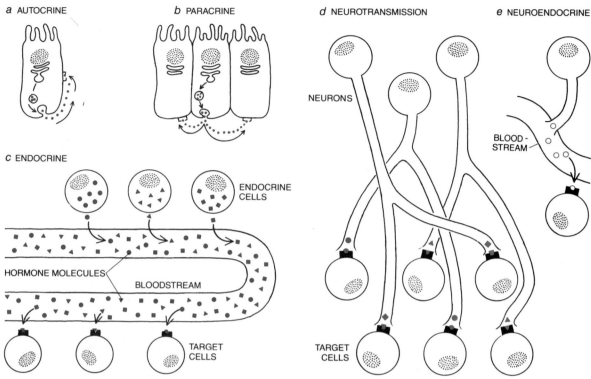

Figure 17 METHODS OF COMMUNICATION of the hormonal and nervous systems. Although autocrine hormones (a) act on the cell that releases them and paracrine hormones (b) act on adjacent cells, most hormones are in the endocrine system and act on cells or organs anywhere in the body. Endocrine glands (c) release hormone molecules into the bloodstream, where they come in contact with receptors on target cells, which recognize the hormone meant to act on that cell and pull them out of the bloodstream. Neurons (d) communicate by releasing neurotransmitters close to target cells. In neuroendocrine action (e) a neuron releases substances that act as hormones directly into the blood.

of cells; neuronal communication can take place in a few milliseconds. In contrast, a hormone released by a particular gland may go on to affect cells or organs in virtually any part of the body; hormonal communication can take several hours.

Yet on the molecular level these two systems are not as dissimilar as they at first seem. Both operate by causing special messenger molecules to come in contact with specific receptors on the target cell. In addition certain neurotransmitters seem, like hormones, to serve only in specialized systems of communication and to perform specific functions.

Recently it has become apparent that there is an even closer relation between the two major systems of intercellular communication: many of the messenger molecules employed by one system are also employed by the other. For instance, norepineph-rine, as a hormone, is released by the adrenal gland to stimulate contractions of the heart, dilate the bronchial tract of the lungs and increase the contractile strength of arm and leg muscles. On the other hand, norepinephrine is also a neurotransmitter: in the sympathetic nervous system it constricts blood vessels, thereby increasing blood pressure.

The same kind of messenger molecule can carry a very different message in the hormonal system than it does in the nervous system. It must be that certain molecules are particularly good mediums of communication.

Molecules that act as hormones generally fall into one of two chemical classes: peptides and steroids. The peptides are strings of amino acids (the subunits of proteins). The steroid hormones are

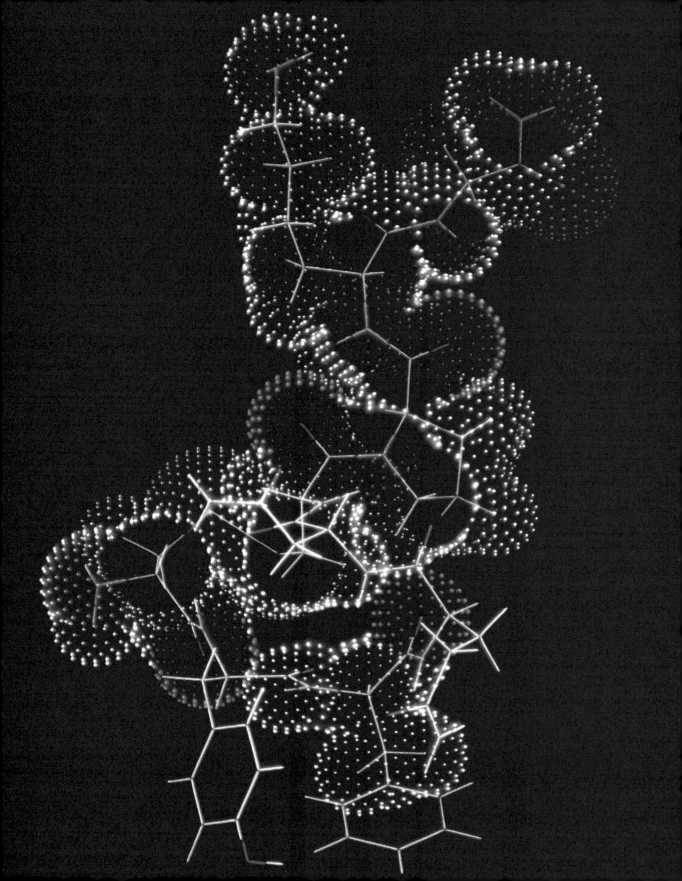

large molecules derived from cholesterol that share the same basic structure: 17 carbon atoms bound together in four closely linked rings (see Figure 19). Small differences in the chemical groups attached to the carbon rings give rise to hormones with quite different functions. Among the major steroid hormones in human beings are the glucocorticoids called cortisol and corticosterone, which regulate the metabolism of glucose and control a wide range of other metabolic functions; the mineral steroids, such as aldosterone, which affect the body's salt balance, and the sex steroids, which include progesterone, testosterone and the estrogen hormones.

The female sex steroids (the estrogens and progesterone) have been characterized more completely than most hormones in the body. They provide an excellent example of how hormones are produced, released and regulated. Estradiol, which is the major estrogen hormone, and progesterone combine during the normal menstrual cycle to prepare the uterus for implantation of a fertilized ovum by building up the uterine wall and increasing blood flow to the uterus. It is an abrupt decline in estradiol and progesterone levels that triggers the bleeding associated with menstruation.

The release of the sex steroids, like that of most hormones, is itself controlled by other hormones and so-called releasing factors from the two master organs: the pituitary and the hypothalamus. Generally speaking, the hypothalamus initiates the release of a steroid hormone from a peripheral gland by releasing a factor that acts on the pituitary. The pituitary then releases other hormones, which act on the peripheral glands. The peripheral glands respond by releasing hormones that act on the target cells.

In the case of the female sex steroids, the major factor released by the hypothalamus is called gonadotropin-releasing hormone. At the beginning of the monthly menstrual cycle the hypothalamus, in-

fluenced by regions of the brain that act as timers, secretes gonadotropin-releasing hormone (which is sometimes called luteinizing-hormone releasing hormone) into the bloodstream. The releasing hormone acts at receptors on the surface of cells within the pituitary that release hormones known as luteinizing hormone and follicle-stimulating hormone.

The follicle-stimulating hormone and to a lesser extent the luteinizing hormone stimulate the growth of small, round follicles in the ovary. The follicles convert cholesterol into estradiol, which they release into the bloodstream. Estradiol goes on to build up muscle tissue in the wall of the uterus. Several days later the pituitary releases a quantity of luteinizing hormone, which changes the structure of the ovarian follicles to form a new entity called the corpus luteum. The transformed follicles synthesize less estradiol and begin to convert cholesterol into progesterone. Progesterone increases blood flow to the uterus and slows the uterine contractions. The combination of estradiol and progesterone has thus prepared the uterine wall to receive a fertilized egg. Soon after ovulation the pituitary begins to release less luteinizing hormone, causing the corpus luteum to stop synthesizing progesterone. Then the cells lining the uterus are sloughed off and menstrual bleeding starts.

Throughout the menstrual cycle the amounts of hormones secreted by various glands must be controlled to ensure that the bloodstream contains the proper concentration of each hormone. This control is achieved through an elaborate set of feedback mechanisms. For example, estradiol released in the ovaries acts not only on its target cells within the uterus but also on the cells in the pituitary that release follicle-stimulating hormone. There it prevents the pituitary from inducing the ovaries to produce more estradiol. Estradiol also acts on the hypothalamus, where it inhibits the release of gonadotropin-releasing hormone. The amount of estradiol in the bloodstream thus determines the additional amount to be released, just as the amount of heat inside a house determines, by way of the thermostat, how much more heat the furnace is to generate.

In the case of estradiol there is another feedback loop as well. When the follicles in the ovaries produce estradiol, they also produce a substance called inhibin. Inhibin acts on both the pituitary and the hypothalamus: in the pituitary it restricts produc-

Figure 18 VASOPRESSIN MOLECULE. As a hormone, vasopressin is released by cells in the posterior pituitary gland. It raises blood pressure by constricting blood vessels and acts as an antidiuretic by increasing the kidneys' ability to reabsorb water. As a neurotransmitter, vasopressin is found in the brain, where it may have a role in memory mechanisms. Solid lines represent bonds between atoms; dotted surfaces delineate the surface of the molecule. Colors show which atoms occupy a region: white for carbon or hydrogen, blue for nitrogen, red for oxygen, orange for phosphorus and yellow for sulfur.

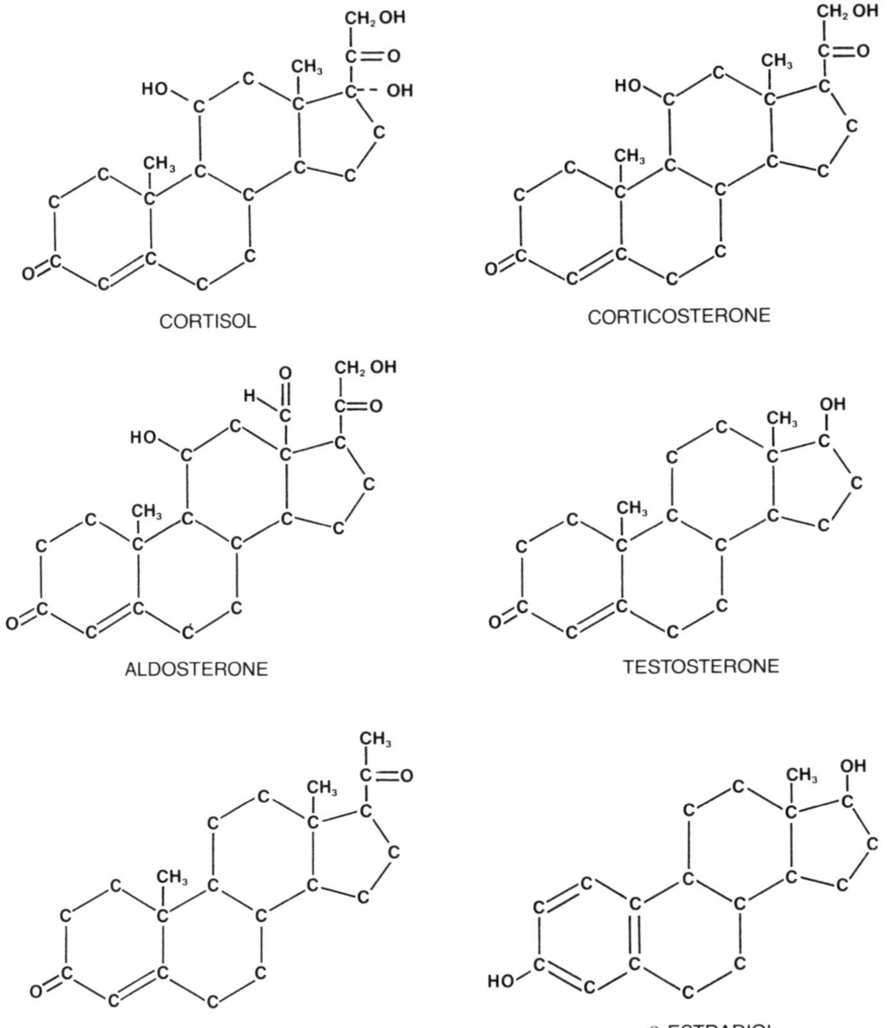

CORTISOL

CORTICOSTERONE

ALDOSTERONE

TESTOSTERONE

PROGESTERONE

β-ESTRADIOL

Figure 19 STEROID HORMONES. The molecules shown represent the primary steroid hormones. Cortisol and corticosterone (glucocorticoids) promote formation of glucose in the liver. Aldosterone enables the kidney to retain so- **dium rather than excreting it in the urine. Testosterone is the principal male sex hormone, and progesterone and estradiol are the major female sex hormones.**

tion of follicle-stimulating hormone, and in the hypothalamus it restricts production of gonadotropin-releasing hormone.

Other steroid hormones, which have widely varying functions, follow similar principles of feedback and control. For instance, the glucocorticoids, such as cortisol, are formed and released when factors and hormones from the hypothalamus and pituitary stimulate the adrenal cortex. Whereas estradiol acts on only a few specific target organs,

cortisol influences nearly every tissue in the body, causing metabolic changes that increase the organism's ability to deal with continuous stress. In most tissues cortisol enhances the uptake and conversion into protein of amino acids, and in the liver it accelerates the conversion of amino acids into sugars. The adrenal cortex is induced to form and secrete cortisol by corticotropin, a hormone synthesized in the pituitary. As Wylie Vale of the Salk Institute for Biological Studies has recently shown, the secretion

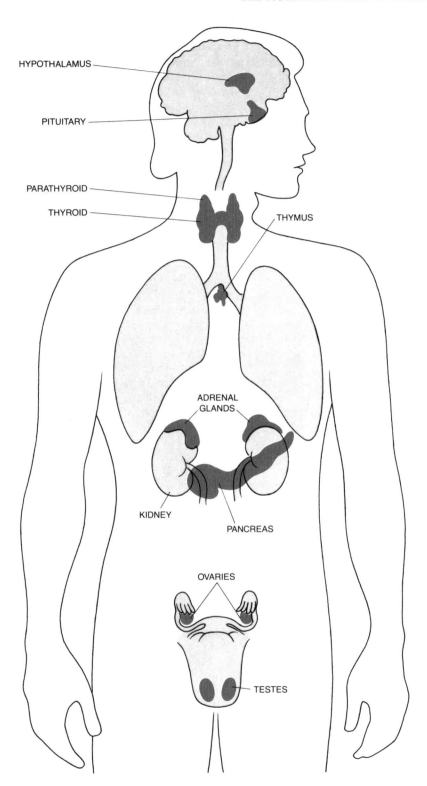

Figure 20 ENDOCRINE SYSTEM consists of several distinct glands and control centers. Endocrine glands are controlled by the pituitary, which secretes hormones that stimulate other glands to synthesize and release their own hormones. The pituitary is controlled by the hypothalamus, which is not a gland but a distinct region of the brain; releasing factors secreted by the hypothalamus control the release of pituitary hormones.

of corticotropin is in turn controlled by the hypothalamus, which secretes a so-called corticotropin-releasing factor.

The hypothalamic releasing factors that regulate the pituitary and the pituitary "master" hormones, which in turn regulate the release of steroid hormones, are themselves not steroids. They are members of the other major chemical class of hormones, the peptide hormones.

Unlike the steroid hormones, which are all synthesized from the same molecule (cholesterol), each peptide hormone derives from a specific "precursor" molecule: a long string of amino acids that contains one or more copies of the hormone as well as other, unrelated peptide sequences. The precursor molecule, which is also called a prohormone, is cleaved by enzymes to release the peptide hormone. Although each peptide hormone is derived from a different precursor, some of the processing enzymes are shared by several systems of peptide hormones.

One of the major peptide hormones is insulin, which is released by specific cells, called the beta cells, in the pancreas. Insulin affects nearly every cell in the body. Although it is best known for lowering the concentration of sugar in the blood by increasing the ability of cells to take up glucose, insulin has many other functions as well, some of which are understood only vaguely. For instance, insulin somehow influences fat metabolism in a way that lowers the concentration of fatty substances circulating in the blood. Hence diabetics, who suffer from insulin deficiency, often develop atherosclerosis, in which plaques of fatty deposits line the blood vessels.

Many of the peptide hormones act in the intestine. Gastrin, for example, is a peptide hormone that stimulates the secretion of acid in the stomach. Patients with gastrin-producing tumors often develop severe ulcers owing to excessive amounts of acid production. Somatostatin is a peptide hormone that counters the effects of gastrin by blocking the secretion of acid at discrete cell groups within the stomach. Another gut peptide, cholesystokinin, is released into the bloodstream by certain cells in the intestine; it travels to the gall bladder, where it increases the flow of bile into the intestine, enhancing digestion.

Cholesystokinin has another function as well: it acts as a neurotransmitter in the brain. Many of the other peptide hormones exhibit the same kind of dual capability, serving as messenger molecules in both hormonal and neural communication. For instance, vasoactive intestinal polypeptide is an intestinal hormone that regulates the motility of the gut, but it is also a brain neurotransmitter. The enkephalins, two peptides that differ slightly from each other, act as opiates in the brain, but in the intestine they are hormones that regulate the movement of food through the digestive pathway by altering the rhythmic peristaltic contractions.

Until the mid-1970's it was not known that peptides could act as neurotransmitters, although many of the peptide hormones were well known. The first neurotransmitters to be identified were acetylcholine, the amines (which are slightly modified chains of amino acids) and the monoamines (modified single amino acids). Examples of monoamines include the catecholamines dopamine, norepinephrine and epinephrine. These three molecules are all derived from the amino acid tyrosine. Norepinephrine and epinephrine (which are also known as noradrenaline and adrenaline) are hormones as well as neurotransmitters; they are released from the adrenal medulla, and they act to increase the heart rate and blood pressure and to increase the flow of sugar into the bloodstream from the liver.

In the 1960's many groups of investigators obtained evidence that a number of unmodified amino acids sometimes serve as neurotransmitters. One such amino acid, gamma-aminobutyric acid, functions almost exclusively as a neurotransmitter. Other amino acid neurotransmitters, such as glutamic acid, aspartic acid and glycine, are constituents of proteins as well.

In all there are no more than 10 neurotransmitters that are amines or amino acids. According to the classical model of neurotransmitter function, any more would be unnecessary. In this model a neurotransmitter acts as a chemical switch that either causes its target neuron to fire or inhibits it from firing. If the model were accurate, the brain would be able to function with only two neurotransmitters, one excitatory and the other inhibitory. Yet since 1975, when it was discovered that the enkephalins are neurotransmitters that act at opiate receptors in the brain, investigators have isolated almost 50 additional "neuropeptides." What do they do?

Careful electrophysiological studies have shown that different neurotransmitters can produce many different effects at synapses. There are a number of different kinds of pores, or channels, in the cell membrane of the target neuron. These channels,

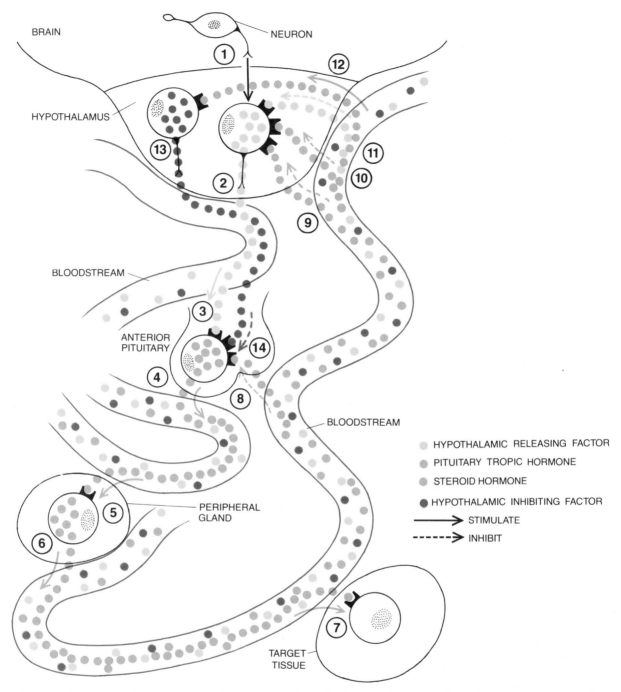

BRAIN

NEURON

HYPOTHALAMUS

BLOODSTREAM

ANTERIOR PITUITARY

BLOODSTREAM

PERIPHERAL GLAND

TARGET TISSUE

HYPOTHALAMIC RELEASING FACTOR

PITUITARY TROPIC HORMONE

STEROID HORMONE

HYPOTHALAMIC INHIBITING FACTOR

STIMULATE

INHIBIT

Figure 21 FEEDBACK AND CONTROL MECHANISMS. When the hypothalamus is stimulated by neurons in the brain (*1*) it secretes a releasing factor (*2*) into the bloodstream. Some molecules of the factor are pulled out of the blood by receptors of cells in the pituitary (*3*) and induce them to secrete a pituitary tropic hormone (*4*), which travels through the blood to a peripheral gland (*5*) and causes the gland to start producing, say, a steroid hormone (*6*), which affects its target tissue (*7*). Feedback loops maintain the correct concentrations of hormones. For example, the hormone acts on the pituitary (*8*) to inhibit production of pituitary tropic hormone and the hypothalamus to limit production of releasing factor (*9*), both of which also inhibit the hypothalamus from producing the releasing factor (*10*, *11*). The steroid hormone (*12*) induces hypothalamus cells to produce an inhibiting factor (*13*), which inhibits release of the pituitary tropic hormone (*14*).

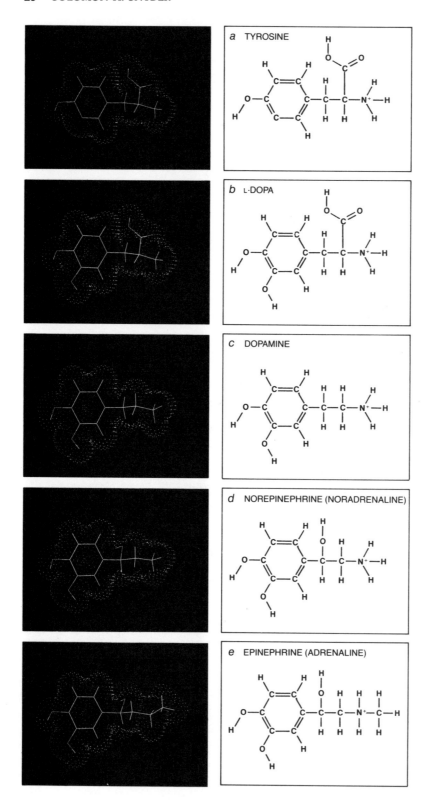

Figure 22 CATECHOLAMINE NEUROTRANSMITTERS. Tyrosine (*a*) is first converted in L-dopa (*b*) by the addition of a hydroxyl (OH) group. Hydrogen replaces a carbon bonded to an OH group and an oxygen to form dopamine (*c*). Adding another OH group yields norepinephrine (*d*), or noradrenaline. Adding a methyl group (CH$_3$) gives epinephrine, or adrenaline (*e*). (Images at left by Tripos Associates.)

which can be opened or closed by a neurotransmitter molecule, allow such ions as chloride, sodium, potassium and calcium to pass through the neuronal membrane. There appear to be many channel types for each ion, and various channels convey different types of electrical information. Neurotransmitters can affect the channels in different ways.

Moreover, a single neurotransmitter may have differing effects depending on the type of synapse at which it is acting. For example, at muscarinic receptors, which are found on smooth-muscle cells in the intestine, the neurotransmitter acetylcholine closes certain channels that normally allow potassium ions to leave the cell. The effect (which is not completely understood) is to produce a gradual, prolonged excitation of the muscle. On the other hand, at nicotinic receptors, which are found on skeletal muscles, acetylcholine opens sodium channels, causing the muscle to contract briskly and rapidly.

In addition to overturning the conception that neurotransmitters deliver only a simple "on" or "off" message, neuropeptides have caused another aspect of traditional thinking to be reconsidered. It had been thought that each neuron releases only a single type of neurotransmitter. In 1977 Tomas G. M. Hökfelt of the Karolinska Institute in Stockholm found that the terminals of many (and perhaps most) neurons contain two or three neurotransmitters. (One of the neurotransmitters is invariably a peptide.) Apparently the "co-transmitters" work together in a synergistic fashion to convey subtler information than would be possible with a single transmitter. It is not yet clear precisely how the mechanisms of co-transmission operate.

M any features of neuropeptides are exemplified by the two enkephalins, which can act as neurotransmitters or as hormones. Both of them are five amino acids long. They differ only in their fifth amino acid: one, called met-enkephalin, ends with methionine and the other, leu-enkephalin, with leucine. Enkephalins are observed in discrete neural pathways throughout the brain in approximately the same areas where opiate receptors are found. The coincidence of the location of enkephalin pathways and opiate receptors supports the hypothesis that the enkephalin neurotransmitters act as opiates.

The enkephalins are synthesized from two large precursor proteins, which are called proenkephalin A and proenkephalin B. Proenkephalin A contains six copies of met-enkephalin and one of leu-enkephalin, whereas proenkephalin B contains three copies of leu-enkephalin and none of met-enkephalin. Hence all met-enkephalin derives from proenkephalin A; leu-enkephalin can be synthesized from either of the two precursors.

Within the precursor molecules each enkephalin is flanked on both sides by two-amino-acid signals: either two lysines or two arginines or one of each. Two successive enzymatic steps are necessary to free enkephalin from the precursor. In the first step an enzyme cuts the peptide bond to the right of each of the flanking amino acids (see Figure 24). The resulting molecule consists of an enkephalin with one extra amino acid attached to the right-hand side. A second enzyme then removes this amino acid to produce enkephalin.

The rate at which enkephalin is formed varies under different circumstances; the rate is thought to accelerate during periods of painful stress. The rate of synthesis can be governed by changes in the rate at which the genes for proenkephalin are transcribed or by the availability of the enzymes that cleave the peptide bonds holding enkephalin within the precursor molecule.

M any enzymes can carry out the two enzymatic steps necessary to convert proenkephalin into enkephalin. One of the most persistent puzzles raised by the neuropeptides has been whether certain generalized enzymes process all hormone and neurotransmitter peptides or whether there are specific enzymes for each peptide. The solution to the puzzle will have profound practical consequences. If specific enzymes are involved, it may be possible to design therapeutic drugs made up of selective enzyme inhibitors that block the biosynthesis of only certain peptide neurotransmitters, allowing precise control over a patient's neurochemistry.

Recent research favors the hypothesis that specialized converting enzymes do indeed exist for each neuropeptide. Lloyd D. Fricker, Stephen M. Strittmatter and David R. Lynch in my laboratory at the Johns Hopkins University School of Medicine have isolated and characterized an enzyme we call enkephalin convertase. It removes the single amino acid that is attached to partially liberated enkephalin. We have found that enkephalin convertase is selectively localized in the same sites in the brain as enkephalin itself, indicating that it contributes to formation of enkephalin in these areas (although it

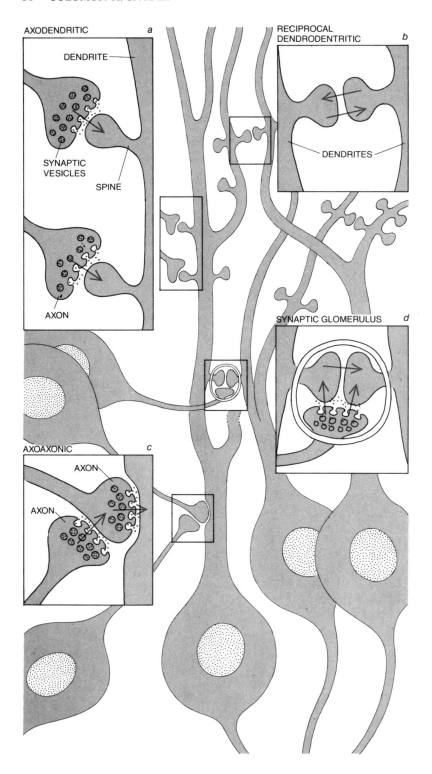

Figure 23   COMMUNICATION BETWEEN NEURONS. In the axodendritic synapse (*a*) synaptic vesicles in the axon of one neuron release neurotransmitter toward receptors on the dendrite of a target neuron. In a reciprocal dendrodendritic synapse (*b*) each dendrite passes messages to the other by way of a separate synapse. In axoaxonic synapses (*c*) the axon of one neuron passes a message through the axon of another neuron to the dendrite of a third neuron. In a synaptic glomerulus (*d*) the axon of one neuron passes messages to dendrites of two others; the dendrites may pass messages to each other as well.

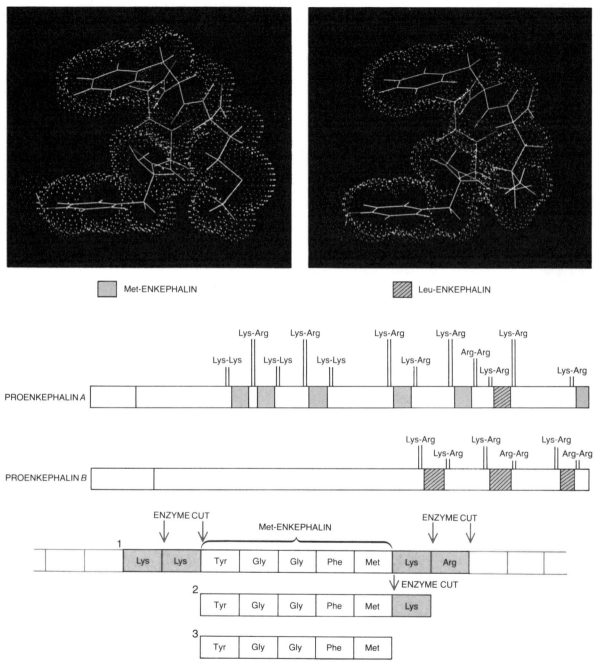

Figure 24 ENKEPHALINS differ only in the fifth amino acid—methionine in met-enkephalin (*top left*) and leucine in leu-enkephalin (*top right*). The two types of enkephalin precursor molecule (*middle*) are proenkephalin A and proenkephalin B. Two enzymes are needed to separate enkephalin from the precursor molecule. The first (*1*) makes a cut to the right of each signaling amino acid (lysine or arginine), leaving an enkephalin molecule with one extra amino acid attached to its right side. The second enzymatic step (*2*) cuts off the extra amino acid to produce enkephalin (*3*). (Images at top by Tripos Associates.)

may have other functions elsewhere in the body). Several drugs we have tested are about 1,000 times more potent at inhibiting enkephalin convertase than any other enzyme.

One of the most exciting consequences of research on neuropeptides, then, is the possibility of developing new drugs that are more effective, more specific and safer than the psychotherapeutic drugs now in use. Virtually every drug used in psychiatry and neurology acts by blocking or enhancing the effects of one or another neurotransmitter. Most drugs exert their effects by acting on one or another of the classical neurotransmitters. The newly discovered peptide transmitters may spawn a new generation of drugs that influence the synthesis, release and receptor effects of specific neuropeptides. With an armamentarium of drugs to regulate each of the many neuropeptides, more precise modulation of feeling and thinking will be possible. The potential for alleviating emotional and neurologic disease will be great.

The ways in which current drugs interact with transmitters are best described by considering norepinephrine, one of the classic amine transmitters. Norepinephrine is a transmitter of the sympathetic nervous system, which is the part of the autonomic nervous system that prepares the body for a rapid expenditure of energy by, for example, dilating certain blood vessels, accelerating the heart rate and slowing digestion. Norepinephrine is also a brain neurotransmitter.

Neurons that contain norepinephrine, like those containing enkephalins, are highly localized in discrete areas of the brain. One of the most prominent norepinephrine pathways is centered in a small nucleus in the brain-stem called the locus coeruleus, from which norepinephrine neurons send axons to many regions of the brain. In this way the relatively few neurons in the locus coeruleus are able to influence literally billions of other neurons.

There are four major types of norepinephrine receptors, called $alpha_1$, $alpha_2$, $beta_1$ and $beta_2$. The different norepinephrine receptors are at differing sites within the body, and so it is possible to design drugs that achieve their effects by blocking or stimulating the effect of norepinephrine at one particular type of receptor. For example, in the peripheral nervous system the stimulation of $alpha_1$ receptors raises blood pressure, and so many drugs for treating hypertension are designed to selectively block $alpha_1$ receptors. Stimulating $beta_1$ or $beta_2$ receptors, on the other hand, speeds the heart rate and dilates the bronchial tree of the lungs. A beta stimulant can therefore be used to treat asthma and a beta blocker to treat angina.

Unfortunately a beta stimulant administered to treat asthma might speed the heart excessively; a beta blocker intended to treat angina could worsen a case of asthma. It is possible to overcome these side effects, however, because the heart has mainly $beta_1$ receptors, whereas the lung has mostly $beta_2$ receptors. Drug designers have therefore been able to use selective $beta_2$ stimulants to relieve the symptoms of asthma without causing cardiac palpitations and $beta_1$ blockers to ease anginal distress without provoking asthma attacks. Many other drugs have been designed that take advantage of the multiplicity of receptor types that exists for most neurotransmitters.

A number of other drugs operate on a slightly different principle. After a neurotransmitter has been released and has acted on receptors, its action must somehow be terminated so that receptors can respond to the next nerve impulse. Most neurotransmitters are inactivated by a pumplike mechanism that transports the neurotransmitter back into the nerve ending from which it was released. Some drugs exert their therapeutic effects by blocking this "reuptake" mechanism. For instance, the major antidepressant drugs, which are called tricyclic antidepressants, block the reuptake inactivation of norepinephrine and serotonin. By inhibiting the norepinephrine and serotonin reuptake systems, the antidepressant drugs make a greater quantity of neurotransmitter available to receptor sites. That such drugs are indeed able to help cure depression indicates that depression may result in part from a deficiency of norepinephrine, serotonin and other biogenic amines (amine transmitters that are produced within the living brain).

Certain other drugs act by influencing the enzymes that synthesize or destroy the norepinephrine molecule. For example, by inhibiting monoamine oxidase, the enzyme that degrades norepinephrine, it is possible to cause a buildup in the levels of norepinephrine in the brain. Much of the accumulated norepinephrine is then forced out of nerve endings by osmotic pressure and acts on receptors. Monoamine oxidase inhibitors can thus increase the synaptic activity of norepinephrine, and so they can be used as antidepressants.

Communication between cells or groups of cells is crucial for the survival of every multicellular organism. In higher organisms the mechanisms of communication rely on a large number of highly specialized messenger molecules. As investigators come to know the properties and functions of all these intercellular messengers, it will become possible to develop safer and more effective therapeutic agents for conditions as diverse as hormonal abnormalities, heart disease and mental illness.

POSTSCRIPT

That hormones and brain active substances are related in a very profound sense has been the dream of many neurochemists. The brain after all cannot be that different from the rest of the organism. However, that the link should end up being as robust as is presently recognized was more than even the most optimistic of researchers ever bargained for. By now a very large number of these bioactive substances have been encountered and their cells of origin have been identified throughout the central and peripheral nervous systems as well as in nonneuronal elements. In fact, the concept of the paracrine neuron introduced by T. Fujita in 1985 epitomizes the close relationship between neurotransmitters and neurohormones. In many ways the next step in the development of this interesting concept is taken up in Chapter 8, "Neuropeptides," by Floyd E. Bloom.

"Second Messengers" in the Brain

Nerve cells communicate by secreting neurotransmitters. These chemical messages are translated by second messengers within the cell into transient and longer-lasting physiological actions.

. . .

James A. Nathanson and Paul Greengard

August, 1977

For a multicellular organism to survive and function effectively its component cells must act in a coordinated fashion. Such coordination necessitates the transfer of information between cells in widely separated parts of the organism, and in most higher animals there are two major pathways of intercellular communication: the endocrine system and the nervous system. In the endocrine system specialized cells secrete hormones, which are carried in the bloodstream to distant parts of the body and influence the activity of specifically responsive target cells. In the nervous system a network of nerve cells with elongated processes communicate with one another by secreting neurotransmitters, which traverse the tiny gap between two nerve cells and produce a change in the electrical activity of the receiving cell.

Both systems involve messenger molecules that are released from one cell, travel a certain distance and interact with the surface of a second cell to modify its activity. In view of this similarity and assuming that nature functions economically one can postulate that some types of chemical transmission between nerve cells might be mediated by mechanisms similar to those mediating the physiological effects of certain hormones. This point of view has led to new perceptions of the biochemical organization of the brain and the mechanism of action of many drugs that affect behavior.

To provide background for a discussion of the molecular mechanisms of nerve transmission, let us first review some current concepts of the mechanism of hormone action. Hormones regulate an enormous range of biochemical processes in their target cells by influencing the rate at which enzymes and other proteins are manufactured, by affecting the activity of enzymes in key metabolic pathways or by altering the permeability of cell membranes. Because these processes operate in the interior of the target cell, the hormone itself or the information conveyed by it must somehow be made available inside the cell.

The delivery of a hormonal message to the interior of the cell appears to be achieved in one of two ways. Steroid hormones, which are derived from cholesterol, are easily soluble in fat and hence can pass through the fatty outer membrane of the target cell and directly influence processes inside it. Hormones of this type include cortisone and the sex hormones estradiol and testosterone. Peptide and amino-acid-derived hormones such as insulin and adrenalin (epinephrine), however, are not able to penetrate the cell membrane because of their size or molecular structure. Instead they attach themselves to specialized receptor sites on the surface of the cell and influence the biochemical machinery from the outside.

The hormone receptors — large protein molecules embedded in the cell membrane — are quite selec-

tive in their ability to bind the hormone for which they were designed, presumably because the molecular configuration of the receptor allows the hormone molecule to fit the receptor quite precisely. The forces that hold the hormone to the receptor are not the covalent ones that bind the atoms in a molecule; they are weaker forces that soon release the hormone, leaving the receptor free to accept additional molecules of the same hormone. Thus the extent to which a hormone influences its target cell depends on the concentration of the hormone in the fluid outside the cell and the affinity of the hormone for the membrane receptor.

Once a hormone has bound to a receptor, how does it convey its message to the interior of the cell? Earl W. Sutherland and his colleagues at Case Western Reserve University first addressed this question some 20 years ago. At that time they were studying the mechanism by which the hormone adrenalin causes liver cells to release the sugar glucose into the bloodstream when the body is under stress. The released glucose comes from the breakdown of glycogen (animal starch), which is held in reserve by the liver. Sutherland and his colleague Theodore W. Rall found that when they exposed to adrenalin cell membranes isolated from liver cells, an unidentified factor was produced that, when it was mixed with the cytoplasm of the liver cells, mimicked the action of adrenalin in causing the conversion of glycogen to glucose. Hence it seemed that the response to the hormone had at least two stages: the interaction of the hormone with the membrane to form the unidentified factor, followed by the factor's activation of the biochemical mechanism in the cytoplasm.

Subsequent experiments identified the factor as cyclic adenosine monophosphate (cyclic AMP), one of the class of small molecules called nucleotides. It is related in structure to adenosine triphosphate (ATP), the universal currency of chemical energy in the cell. The "cyclic" in cyclic AMP refers to the fact that the single phosphate group (PO_4) in the molecule forms a ring with the carbon atoms to which it is attached.

Sutherland and his co-workers soon found that the membranes of liver cells (and many other cells) contain an enzyme, adenylate cyclase, that converts ATP into cyclic AMP. Because ATP is located almost exclusively in the cytoplasm, Sutherland and his colleagues G. Alan Robison and Reginald W. Butcher reasoned that at least part of the adenylate

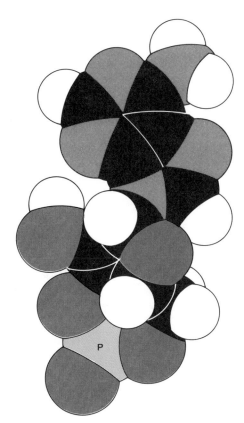

● CARBON

◍ OXYGEN

◍ NITROGEN

○ HYDROGEN

Ⓟ PHOSPHORUS

Figure 25 SPACE-FILLING MODEL of cyclic AMP shows that the molecule is compact. It consists of a five-carbon sugar to which are attached an adenine ring (*top*) and a phosphate group.

cyclase molecule must face inward and that the cyclic AMP manufactured by the enzyme is released into the interior of the cell. When they exposed liver cells to adrenalin, the rate at which adenylate cyclase converted ATP into cyclic AMP was substantially increased, indicating that there was a functional link between the binding of hormone to the receptor on the outside of the membrane and the activation of adenylate cyclase on the inside. Such a connection was subsequently shown to exist for a wide variety of hormones that bind to membrane receptors, although since different kinds of cells possess receptors for different hormones, a given hormone will increase the level of cyclic AMP in its target cells but not in other cells.

It is now generally accepted that the cyclic AMP generated by adenylate cyclase in response to the binding of a hormone to the receptor acts as a "second messenger" to relay the message of the hormone (the first messenger) from the membrane to the cell's biochemical machinery. In this way the low-level signal represented by the hormone can be amplified many thousands of times by the manufacture of cyclic AMP.

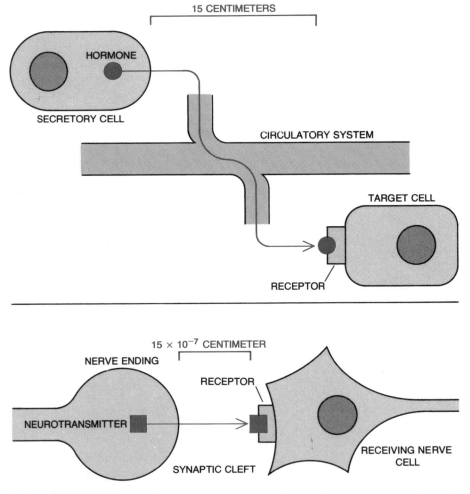

Figure 26 ANALOGOUS MECHANISMS underlie communication in the endocrine system (*top*) and the nervous system (*bottom*). In both chemical messengers (respectively hormones and neurotransmitters) are released from one cell, travel through the extracellular medium and bind to receptors on the surface of a second cell to modify its activity. The intracellular effects of many hormones and neurotransmitters appear to be mediated by the second-messenger cyclic AMP.

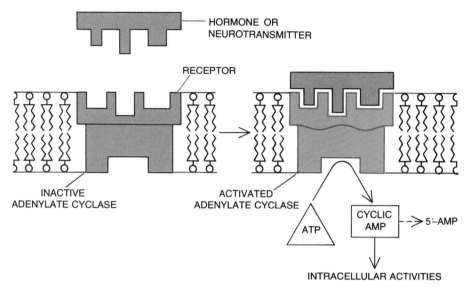

Figure 27 ADENYLATE CYCLASE IS ACTIVATED by the binding of a hormone or a neurotransmitter to its receptor on the cell membrane. The enzyme then converts some of the ATP in the cytoplasm into cyclic AMP, which relays the signal from the membrane to interior of the cell.

U p to this point we have discussed the interactions among hormones, receptors and cyclic AMP in cells outside the nervous system. Can analogous mechanisms help to explain how nerve cells communicate? The nerve cell, or neuron, is the basic structural and functional unit of the central nervous system; behavior is the net result of the complex interaction of many nerve cells. Information is conveyed along the elongated fiber of a neuron in the form of an electrochemical impulse. The impulse stops, however, when it reaches the tiny synapse, or gap, that separates the fiber terminal from its receiving neuron. To bridge the synapse and reinitiate electrochemical transmission, neurotransmitter is released and travels across the gap between one cell and the next. Like the hormones we have been discussing, neurotransmitters do not enter the receiving cell but interact with receptors on the outside of the cell membrane, leading to a change in the electric potential across the membrane.

The first connection between cyclic AMP and brain function was made when Sutherland and his co-workers found a large amount of the enzyme adenylate cyclase in the brain of vertebrate animals, indicating that cyclic AMP was being actively manufactured there. In 1967 Eduardo De Robertis, working in collaboration with Butcher and Sutherland, found that when brain tissue was disrupted by homogenization and the resulting subcellular components were separated according to their density by spinning them in a centrifuge, those fractions containing the largest amount of pinched-off nerve endings also showed the highest level of adenylate cyclase activity. This finding was interesting because many of the nerve-ending particles include fragments of membrane from both sides of the synaptic junction and hence represent the precise areas of the brain where nerve cells communicate. The fact that adenylate cyclase was specifically associated with those areas suggested that cyclic AMP might somehow be involved in synaptic transmission.

In the same experiments it was found that the nerve-ending particles also contained high levels of phosphodiesterase, an enzyme that degrades cyclic AMP into a physiologically inactive form of adenosine monophosphate. Somewhat later Noel T. Florendo and Russell J. Barrnett, working in collaboration with our laboratory at the Yale University School of Medicine, developed a cytochemical procedure to determine the location of phosphodiesterase within individual cells with the aid of the electron microscope. Using this technique, they demonstrated that the phosphodiesterase activity in

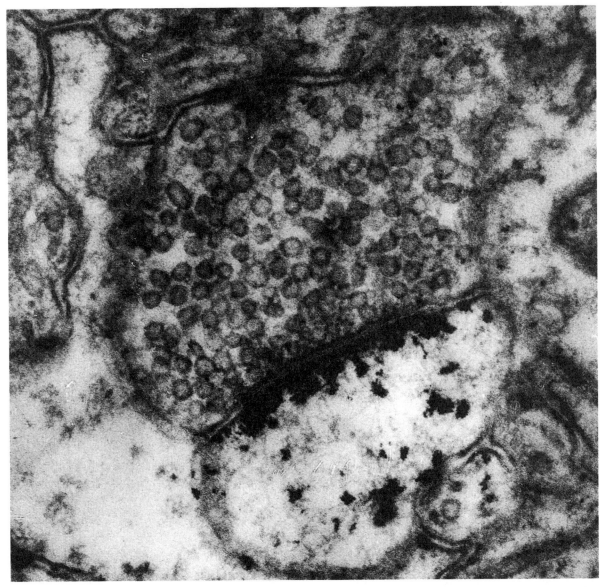

Figure 28 LOCALIZATION OF PHOSPHODIESTERASE was accomplished by applying chemicals to brain tissue that reacted with the enzyme's product to form a dense precipitate. In this micrograph of a single synaptic junction the precipitate marking the location of phosphodiesterase is associated with the region of the receiving cell membrane possessing neurotransmitter receptors, supporting the hypothesis that the neurotransmitter molecules released from the circular vesicles in the nerve terminal (*top*) bind to the receptors and induce the manufacture of cyclic AMP.

the synaptic region was localized in the part of the membrane of the receiving cell thought to possess neurotransmitter receptors. This localization further suggested a role for cyclic AMP in synaptic transmission, since phosphodiesterase at the postsynaptic site would have access to, and hence be able to degrade, cyclic AMP that had been synthesized as a result of the stimulation of adenylate cyclase by a neurotransmitter.

At about this time several experiments demonstrated that electrical or neurotransmitter-induced stimulation of nerve tissue could result in large increases in cyclic AMP. In our laboratory Donald A. McAfee and Michel Schorderet, working with a sympathetic-nervous-system ganglion from the neck of rabbits and cattle, showed that electrical stimulation of the nerves innervating the ganglion, resulting in synaptic transmission, was associated with an elevation in cyclic AMP levels. McAfee and John W. Kebabian then showed that the application

of the neurotransmitter dopamine to these ganglia mimicked the effect of electrical stimulation in elevating cyclic AMP levels, and conversely that the application of cyclic AMP could reproduce some of the electrophysiological effects of dopamine. Meanwhile Shiro Kakiuchi and Rall at Case Western Reserve, and somewhat later John W. Daly and his co-workers at the National Institute of Arthritis,

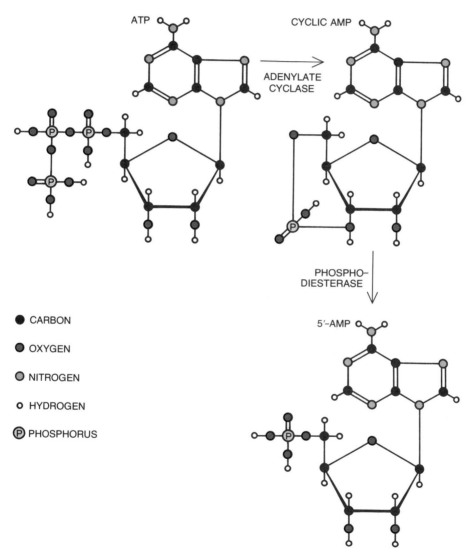

Figure 29 SYNTHESIS AND DEGRADATION of cyclic AMP are accomplished by two enzymes associated with the outer membrane of certain hormone-sensitive and neurotransmitter-sensitive cells. Adenylate cyclase converts ATP into cyclic AMP by removing two phosphate groups from the molecule's carbon backbone to form a ring. Phosphodiesterase inactivates cyclic AMP by opening the phosphate ring, converting the molecule into an inert form of AMP.

Metabolism, and Digestive Diseases, reported that chopped pieces of brain tissue show large increases in cyclic AMP content when they are exposed to solutions containing various neurotransmitters such as norepinephrine or histamine.

Although all these experiments indicated that there was some kind of association between neurotransmitter receptors and cyclic AMP levels, they left unanswered the question of whether the effects of any particular neurotransmitter were coupled directly to the activation of adenylate cyclase. In order to prove a functional link between the binding of a particular neurotransmitter to its receptor and the subsequent synthesis of cyclic AMP it was necessary to demonstrate the presence of a specific neurotransmitter-sensitive adenylate cyclase, that is, an enzyme whose activity is largely dependent on the presence of a particular neurotransmitter. Before describing this enzyme in more detail it is worth discussing briefly how a neurotransmitter receptor is linked to the action of drugs that affect behavior.

Since nerve cells communicate primarily by releasing neurotransmitters at synaptic junctions, it follows that anything that interferes with the binding of a neurotransmitter to its receptor will disrupt normal nerve-cell communication and thereby alter behavior. Such interference can be produced by foreign substances, for example drugs, that have been introduced into the bloodstream. If a particular drug has a molecular configuration similar to that of a native neurotransmitter, it may be able to bind to the membrane receptor for that neurotransmitter and mimic the neurotransmitter's action. Drugs of this type are called receptor agonists. If the drug has a configuration similar to that of a neurotransmitter but not quite as similar as that of a receptor agonist, it may be able to bind to the receptor without activating it. In that case the drug will prevent the activation of the receptor by a neurotransmitter. Drugs of this type are called receptor antagonists. Other drugs that influence behavior are neither agonists nor antagonists. Some may have a mixed action by binding to the neurotransmitter receptor and causing partial activation; some may affect the receptor indirectly by altering the amount of neurotransmitter available for binding. Over the past several years this relatively simple concept of the relations among drugs, receptors and behavior has led to substantial advances in our understanding and treatment of disorders of the nervous system and has focused attention on the role cyclic AMP may play in both normal and abnormal brain function.

For example, it is generally accepted that the symptoms of Parkinson's disease, or shaking palsy, result from the degeneration of a group of neurons whose fibers project to the basal ganglia near the center of the brain from a region at the base of the brain known as the substantia nigra. These neurons secrete the neurotransmitter dopamine at their fiber terminals, and their degeneration reduces the amount of dopamine available to interact with the receptors on the receiving cells in the basal ganglia. As a result the receiving cells begin to function abnormally and cause the symptoms characteristic of Parkinson's disease: tremor, rigidity and a delay in the initiation of movement. Although dopamine is depleted in the brains of patients with the disease, the dopamine receptors in the basal ganglia appear to be undamaged.

These facts, set forth in large part by Arvid Carlsson of the University of Göteborg, Oleh Hornykiewicz of the University of Vienna and the late George C. Cotzias of the Brookhaven National Laboratory, have led to a dramatic new treatment for Parkinson's disease: the administration of the drug levo-dihydroxyphenylalanine (L-dopa), the amino acid precursor of dopamine. When L-dopa is given orally, it enters the bloodstream and travels to the brain, where it is taken up and converted to dopamine. (The neurotransmitter itself cannot enter the brain from the circulation.) The newly manufactured dopamine can then act as an agonist: it stimulates the dopamine receptors in the basal ganglia. By making up for the lack of native dopamine in this way, L-dopa is able to reverse some of the symptoms of the disease.

Drugs that act as antagonists of the dopamine receptor are also of therapeutic value. Such drugs include the phenothiazine tranquilizer chlorpromazine (Thorazine), which is widely used in the treatment of schizophrenia. Psychotic patients treated with chlorpromazine often show a dramatic improvement in their mental symptoms, but the side effects of the drug limit its clinical usefulness. For example, after prolonged treatment patients may begin to manifest tremors and other abnormal movements similar to those seen in Parkinson's disease. When administration of the tranquilizer is stopped, the abnormal movements usually disappear. Hence it seems that chlorpromazine brings on a drug-induced Parkinson's disease by blocking dopamine receptors in the basal ganglia, thereby mimicking the symptoms of dopamine depletion even

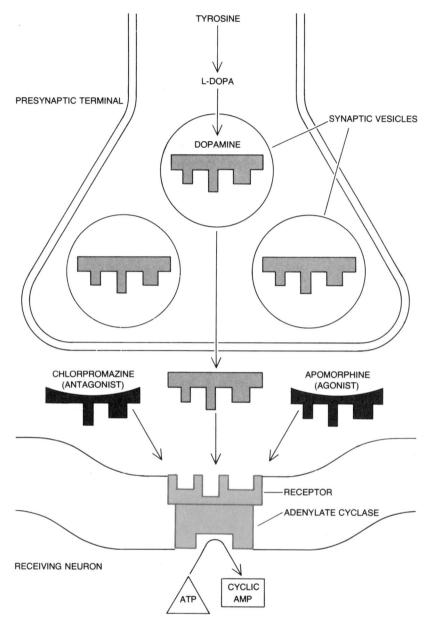

Figure 30 DOPAMINE released by the activity of presynaptic nerve terminals traverses the synaptic space and binds to a postsynaptic dopamine receptor, resulting in the activation of adenylate cyclase and the synthesis of cyclic AMP within the postsynaptic cell. The activity of the dopamine-sensitive adenlyate cyclase is influenced by drugs known to bind specifically to dopamine receptors. Antagonist drugs such as chlorpromazine block the receptor and prevent its activation by dopamine. Agonist drugs such as apomorphine mimic the action of dopamine by activating the receptor.

though normal amounts of the neurotransmitter may be present.

Besides being a troublesome side effect of antipsychotic drug treatment, drug-induced Parkinson's disease has shed some light on the biochemical abnormalities that may underlie schizophrenia. If drugs that appear to block dopamine receptors alleviate the symptoms of schizophrenia, then perhaps schizophrenia results from an overactivity of dopamine-containing neurons in certain parts of the brain. The overactivity of these cells would cause an excessive release of dopamine from their nerve endings, leading to an overstimulation of postsynaptic dopamine receptors. By blocking these receptors chlorpromazine apparently prevents this overstimulation and so diminishes the symptoms of schizophrenia.

These two findings—that dopamine-receptor agonists are useful agents against Parkinson's disease and that dopamine-receptor antagonists are effective agents against schizophrenia—made it highly desirable to further understand the biochemical nature of the dopamine receptor in the brain of mammals. The work of Kebabian, McAfee and Schorderet described above had suggested that cyclic AMP might play an important role in mediating neuronal responses to dopamine. In order to show that neurotransmitter binding and cyclic AMP synthesis were functionally linked, however, it was necessary to identify an adenylate cyclase that would synthesize cyclic AMP from ATP in the presence of dopamine.

In 1972 Kebabian, together with Gary L. Petzold of our laboratory, obtained experimental evidence demonstrating the presence of a dopamine-sensitive adenylate cyclase in the caudate nucleus, one of the basal ganglia of the brain and a region rich in dopamine receptors. The enzyme was located in synaptic membranes and bore a remarkable similarity to the dopamine receptor. Its activity was stimulated by very low concentrations of dopamine and was strongly inhibited by two classes of antischizophrenic drugs known to block the dopamine receptor. These results strongly suggested that the dopamine receptor in the caudate nucleus and in certain other areas of the mammalian brain might in fact be a component of the dopamine-sensitive adenylate cyclase, and that cyclic AMP might therefore mediate the intracellular action of dopamine at certain synapses.

Further investigations by Yvonne Clement-Cormier and Kebabian in our laboratory and by Leslie L. Iversen and his co-workers at the University of Cambridge have largely confirmed that suggestion: among a large number of substances there is a remarkable parallel between the ability to act as an agonist or antagonist of the dopamine receptor and the ability to activate or inhibit the dopamine-sensitive adenylate cyclase. This correlation has since led to a new methodology for the rapid screening and development of drugs as potential dopamine receptor agonists (agents against Parkinson's disease) or antagonists (agents against schizophrenia). Whereas the traditional methods of measuring dopamine receptor activity involved behavioral tests that were time-consuming and often imprecise, the determination of the activity of the dopamine-sensitive adenylate cyclase in the presence of the drug under investigation provides a rapid and quantitative way of evaluating the drug's ability to either block or activate the dopamine receptor.

A link between cyclic AMP and synaptic transmission was also indicated when Floyd E. Bloom, Barry Hoffer and George Siggins, working at the National Institute of Mental Health, found physiological evidence that some of the actions of the neurotransmitter norepinephrine are mediated by cyclic AMP. At that time Bloom and his colleagues were studying the regulation by norepinephrine of neuronal activity in the cerebellum, which controls many of the automatic movements of the body, such as walking. The key elements that regulate such movements are large, elaborately branching neurons called Purkinje cells found in the cortex, or outer layer, of the cerebellum. Extending earlier anatomical work by Tomas Hokfelt and Kjell Fuxe at the Karolinska Institute in Stockholm, Bloom and his colleagues found that the locus coeruleus, a small cluster of norepinephrine-containing neurons buried deep in the brain stem, sends fine connections to the cortex of the cerebellum, and that stimulation of this pathway causes the firing rate of the Purkinje cells to decrease markedly. When they administered measured amounts of norepinephrine or cyclic AMP to individual Purkinje cells with a micropipette, they observed that the application of either compound slowed the firing rate of these cells in the same way that stimulation of the locus coeruleus did. Moreover, by means of a fluorescent-labeling technique that stains selectively for cyclic AMP they were able to show that either stimulation of the locus coeruleus or the direct application of norepinephrine causes a dramatic increase in the cyclic AMP content of the Purkinje cells. These and other results have suggested that the effects of norepinephrine on Purkinje-cell firing are mediated through the stimulation of a norepinephrine-sensitive adenylate cyclase and the resulting synthesis of cyclic AMP inside the cell.

Recent experiments in our laboratory have indicated that the role of cyclic AMP in the functioning of neurotransmitter receptors is by no means limited to the nervous system of vertebrates. For example, we have found in the thoracic ganglia of insects an enzyme that may mediate the effects of the neurotransmitter serotonin. This serotonin-sensitive adenylate cyclase is activated by very low concentrations of serotonin, and the effect of serotonin on the activity of the enzyme is specifically inhibited by drugs that are known to block serotonin receptors. Interestingly enough, one of the most potent of these blocking agents is the hallucinogen lysergic acid diethylamide (LSD). Our findings suggest that the serotonin receptor of neural tissue is intimately associated with a serotonin-sensitive adenylate cyclase and that some of the physiological effects of LSD may result from the inhibition of the enzyme.

At least five neurotransmitters have now been shown to stimulate specific neurotransmitter-sensitive adenylate cyclases: dopamine, norepinephrine, serotonin, histamine and octopamine. Moreover, recently acquired evidence suggests that a second cyclic nucleotide, cyclic guanosine monophosphate (cyclic GMP), may be involved in the effects of the neurotransmitter acetylcholine at certain synapses through the activation of guanylate cyclase, an enzyme that converts guanosine triphosphate (GTP) into cyclic GMP. Cyclic GMP may also be involved in mediating the effects of norepinephrine and histamine at certain receptors that are distinct from those associated with the cyclic AMP system.

It is worth noting that many of the behavioral drugs that affect neurotransmitter receptors produce effects resembling those that occur naturally in patients with mental or neurological diseases. For example, miners exposed to manganese poisoning or patients given antischizophrenic drugs exhibit a syndrome indistinguishable from naturally occurring Parkinson's disease, and LSD can produce hallucinations similar to those experienced by schizophrenics. These and other clinical observations raise the possibility that certain neurological and mental diseases may result from abnormalities in specific receptor-adenylate-cyclase systems. Such abnormalities might arise genetically through nonlethal mutations or be acquired through exposure to high levels of environmental toxins such as manganese.

Not all neurotransmitter receptors, however, have been linked to the synthesis of a cyclic nucleotide. For example, one of the best-studied synaptic mechanisms—the stimulation of the contraction of voluntary muscle through the release of acetylcholine at the junction between a nerve fiber and a muscle—appears to operate independently of the synthesis of a cyclic nucleotide [see "The Response to Acetylcholine," by Henry A. Lester; SCIENTIFIC AMERICAN, February, 1977]. This makes sense in view of the fact that the mediation of synaptic transmission by cyclic nucleotides involves a complex series of steps, which we shall discuss, that makes the process relatively long-lasting on the time scale of neuronal events. Those types of transmission that place a premium on speed, such as the contraction of voluntary muscle, therefore rely on faster receptor mechanisms.

So far we have described how certain neurotransmitters, by binding to a specific receptor, stimulate the production of cyclic AMP inside the receiving cell. The question remains: How does an increase in the level of cyclic AMP translate the message of the neurotransmitter into physiological action?

We know from the work of many neurobiologists over the past 20 years that a nerve cell responds to synaptic stimulation with a brief change in the permeability of the synaptic membrane to one or more kinds of ion. This change in permeability allows ions to flow across the membrane, generating an electric current and thereby altering the membrane's electric potential, or voltage (see Figure 32). Depending on the ions that move and the direction of their movement, the change in electric potential induced by a neurotransmitter will make it either more or less likely that the cell will reach the threshold of excitation necessary for it to generate an impulse. In this respect a neuron acts much like an analogue computer, integrating the many hundreds of inhibitory and excitatory chemical messages that impinge on its surface at any given moment before deciding whether or not to fire.

In order to explore the possible role of cyclic AMP in mediating some of the changes in membrane permeability induced by neurotransmitters, we began several years ago a detailed investigation of the chain of biochemical events that occur inside a neuron following the binding of a neurotransmitter to its receptor and the activation of adenylate cyclase. Earlier experiments by Edwin G. Krebs and his colleagues at the University of Washington had provided some important clues. In their investigation of the mechanism by which adrenaline induces the conversion of glycogen into glucose in muscle cells, they found that the cyclic AMP generated inside the cells by the hormone-sensitive adenylate cyclase caused the transfer of a phosphate group from ATP to the enzyme responsible for the initiation of glycogen breakdown. Somewhat later they discovered that the actual transfer of the phosphate group, the process called phosphorylation, was accomplished by the enzyme protein kinase. In biochemical nomenclature, kinase (more properly, phosphokinase) is a term reserved for enzymes that transfer a phosphate group from ATP to another molecule; for a protein kinase the other molecule is always a protein.

Cyclic AMP is thought to activate protein kinase by binding to an inhibitory subunit of the kinase in such a way as to change its shape and cause it to dissociate from the rest of the enzyme. The loss of the inhibitory component enhances the activity of the kinase, which then readily transfers a phosphate group to the enzyme controlling the pathway of glycogen breakdown. The addition of a phosphate group to this enzyme causes it to trigger a "cascade" of enzymatic reactions, leading ultimately to the breakdown of glycogen. Protein kinase therefore acts as the link between the cyclic AMP generated by the hormone and the activation of the biochemical pathway that accounts for the hormone's metabolic effects.

On the basis of this scheme we began looking for an analogous system in brain cells. Although glycogen breakdown is not a prominent effect of cyclic AMP in nervous tissue, we felt that a similar protein kinase could translate the change in cyclic AMP levels brought about by a neurotransmitter into a change in the permeability of the postsynaptic membrane to ions.

Within a relatively short time J.-F. Kuo and Eishichi Miyamoto, working in our laboratory, isolated a cyclic-AMPa-dependent protein kinase from cattle brain. The enzyme was present in relatively large amounts in the brain tissue compared with most other tissues, and its activity was notably dependent on the presence of cyclic AMP. Furthermore, the concentration of cyclic AMP required to stimulate the enzyme to half its maximum activity was similar to the concentration of cyclic AMP normally found in brain tissue. This finding indicated that the increases in cyclic AMP levels known to be induced by various neurotransmitters would cause large changes in the activity of the cyclic-AMP-dependent protein kinase.

Other experiments demonstrated that the protein kinase could transfer a phosphate group to proteins other than those associated with the breakdown of glycogen. In fact, studies by Hiroo Maeno and Edward Johnson in our laboratory indicated that when brain tissue was homogenized, the proteins phosphorylated to the greatest extent were in the fractions of the homogenized tissue with the largest amounts of synaptic-membrane fragments, and that these fractions also had the greatest concentration of protein kinase.

Thus it became evident that the synaptic membrane contains all the major elements for the neuro-

NEUROTRANSMITTER	TYPE OF RECEPTOR
DOPAMINE	dopamine
NOREPINEPHRINE	alpha-adrenergic
	beta-adrenergic
SEROTONIN	serotonin
HISTAMINE	H_1
	H_2
ACETYLCHOLINE	muscarinic (slow)
	nicotinic (fast).
ENKEPHALIN	opiate

Figure 31 DRUGS AFFECTING BEHAVIOR either interact directly with the neurotransmitter receptor or affect the receptor indirectly by altering the amount of neurotransmitter available for binding. Drugs affecting neurotrans-

transmitter-induced transfer of a phosphate group to a substrate protein in the membrane: (1) a neurotransmitter-sensitive adenylate cyclase that generates cyclic AMP in response to a specific neurotransmitter, (2) a cyclic-AMP-dependent protein kinase that phosphorylates a substrate protein in the presence of cyclic AMP and (3) the membrane substrate protein that is phosphorylated by the protein kinase. The transfer of a phosphate group to such a protein could conceivably change the permeability of the membrane to ions, either directly by changing the configuration of the protein in order to open a channel that ions can flow through, or indirectly, for example by affecting the activity of an enzyme "pump" that physically transports ions across the membrane.

Further investigation showed that the synaptic-membrane fractions also contain the enzymatic ma-

EVIDENCE FOR MEDIATION BY A CYCLIC NUCLEOTIDE		DRUGS ACTING AT THE NEUROTRANSMITTER RECEPTOR		DRUGS AFFECTING THE LEVEL OF NEUROTRANSMITTER AVAILABLE TO THE RECEPTOR	
CYCLIC AMP	CYCLIC GMP	AGONISTS (ACTIVATE RECEPTOR)	ANTAGONISTS (BLOCK RECEPTOR)	INCREASE LEVELS	DECREASE LEVELS
yes	no	apomorphine alpha-bromcryptine	antischizophrenics (Thorazine, Haldol)	levo-dihydroxyphenylalanine (L-DOPA) amantadine amphetamines (Dexedrine) methylphenidate (Ritalin)	alpha-methyl-para-tyrosine
no	yes (?)	phenylephrine (Neosynephrine)	phentolamine (Regitine)	tricyclic antidepressants (Elavil, Tofranil) MAO inhibitors (Parnate) amphetamines cocaine	reserpine (Serpasil) alpha-methyl-dopa (Aldomet)
yes	no	epinephrine (adrenalin) isoproterenol (Isuprel)	propranolol (Inderal)		
yes	no	5-methoxy-N,N-dimethyltryptamine	lysergic acid diethylamide (LSD) methysergide (Sansert)	tricyclic antidepressants (Elavil, Anafranil) tryptophan	para-chloro-phenylalanine
no	yes (?)	2-methyl-histamine	diphenhydramine (Benadryl) dimenhydrinate (Dramamine)	histidine amodiaquine	alpha-hydrazino-histidine brocresine
yes	no	betazole (Histalog)	metiamide cimetidine		
no	yes (?)	pilocarpine carbachol bethanechol (Urecholine)	scopolamine atropine (belladonna) propantheline (Pro-Banthine)	insecticides (Parathion, Malathion) nerve gas (DFP) pyridostigmine (Mestinon)	botulinus toxin
no	no	nicotine	d-tubocurarine (curare) succinylcholine (Anectine)		
yes	?	morphine heroin methadone meperidine (Demerol)	naloxone (Narcan)		

mitter levels work in various ways, such as increasing the synthesis of a neurotransmitter (L-dopa), inducing the release of preexisting neurotransmitter (amphetamine) or blocking the breakdown or sequestration of neurotransmitter levels work in various ways, such as increasing the release of preexisting neurotransmitter (amphetamine) or blocking the breakdown or sequestration of neurotransmitter (certain antidepressants). Cyclic AMP and a related compound, cyclic GMP, appear to mediate the actions of several neurotransmitters and to play a role in the action of many behavioral drugs.

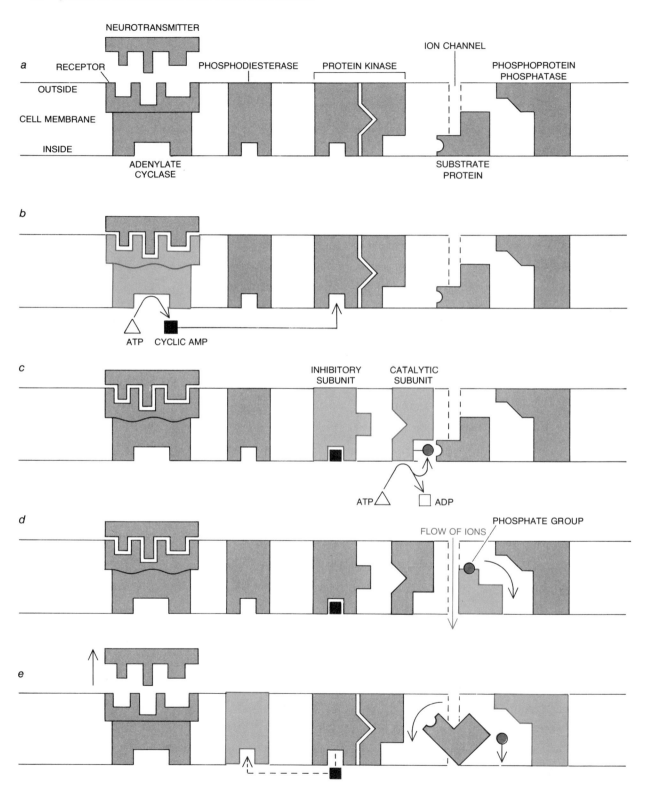

chinery necessary for stopping the cyclic-AMP-dependent phosphorylation process and restoring the membrane to its resting state. These enzymes include not only phosphodiesterase, which degrades cyclic AMP to an inactive form of AMP, but also phosphoprotein phosphatase, which removes the phosphate group from proteins that have previously been phosphorylated by the cyclic-AMP-dependent protein kinase. Several of the components of this membrane-bound enzyme system have been shown to exist as a complex, thereby reducing the distance reaction products must travel from one enzyme to the next and enabling a phosphate group to be rapidly added to and removed from the substrate protein.

Following the discovery that fractions of homogenized brain tissue containing the largest amounts of synaptic membrane serve as excellent substrates for the cyclic-AMP-dependent protein kinase, Tetsufumi Ueda, Bruce K. Krueger and Javier Forn of our laboratory, together with Johnson and Maeno, attempted to isolate the specific protein or proteins that were being phosphorylated. Up to this point it had not been possible to tell whether a large percentage or only a very few of the dozens of proteins known to be present in the synaptic membrane were acting as substrates for phosphorylation. When Ueda and his co-workers incubated synaptic-membrane fractions in a solution containing radioactively labeled ATP in the presence or absence of cyclic AMP, they found that the phosphorylation of only two or three of the several dozen proteins in the membrane fraction was markedly increased by cyclic AMP. This result was gratifying, since it indicated that the effects of cyclic AMP on the phosphorylation of synaptic-membrane protein were specific and did not simply involve a general stimulation of cellular metabolism (see Figure 33).

One of the synaptic-membrane proteins specifically phosphorylated by the cyclic-AMP-dependent protein kinase, designated Protein I, has recently been investigated in detail in our laboratory. Protein I, which has two molecular subunits, Ia and Ib, is localized almost exclusively in the synaptic region of nerve tissue and is apparently absent from those organelles of nerve cells (such as nuclei, mitochondria and ribosomes) that are not directly associated with synaptic transmission. Moreover, Protein I has not been found at all in any non-neuronal tissue (such as heart or liver) yet examined. It is also absent from the brain of fetal rats at stages of development before the formation of connections between nerve cells, and it appears for the first time at the stage when synaptic complexes form.

The phosphorylation of Protein I by protein kinase in the synaptic membrane is extremely fast. In fact, in the shortest period that has yet been accurately studied — five seconds — the phosphorylation is already at the maximum level. The speed of this reaction is virtually a prerequisite to seriously considering the possibility that Protein I might be involved in the generation of the very brief changes in the permeability of the synaptic membrane to ions (lasting for a few hundred milliseconds or less) that give rise to postsynaptic potentials.

If protein phosphorylation mediated by cyclic AMP is indeed responsible for changes in the permeability of the synaptic membrane to ions, then there should be a correlation between the state of phosphorylation of a particular membrane protein or proteins and the state of ion permeability of the cell membrane. The short duration of changes in the permeability of membranes in the nervous system has made it difficult to establish such a correlation within the limitations of present methodology. For this reason we have turned to some non-neuronal model systems, including the red blood cell of the turkey and the frog, to study such permeability changes in detail. Under appropriate conditions these cells respond to hormones such as adrenalin with an increase in the movement of sodium and potassium ions across the cell membrane. This increase, which is due to a change in membrane permeability, appears to be mediated by cyclic AMP.

Recently Stephen A. Rudolph of our laboratory has found that a single large membrane protein becomes phosphorylated whenever cyclic AMP or the adrenalin-related drug isoproterenol is added to

Figure 32 INCREASE IN CYCLIC AMP. The molecular components in the process are shown in their resting state (*a*). When an electrical impulse reaches the presynaptic terminal, neurotransmitter is released, crosses the synaptic space and binds to receptors on the cell, activating adenylate cyclase to convert ATP into cyclic AMP (*b*), which binds to the inhibitory subunit of protein kinase, causing it to dissociate from the catalytic subunit. Now activated, the catalytic subunit transfers a phosphate group from ATP to a substrate protein (*c*). Phosphate changes the shape or position of the substrate protein, allowing certain ions to flow through existing pores in the membrane and altering the electrical excitability of the cell (*d*). The neurotransmitter dissociates from the receptor, stopping further synthesis of cyclic AMP. Phosphodiesterase rapidly inactivates the remaining supply. Finally, phosphoprotein phosphatase removes phosphate group from the substrate protein (*e*).

MINUS CYCLIC
AMP

PLUS CYCLIC
AMP

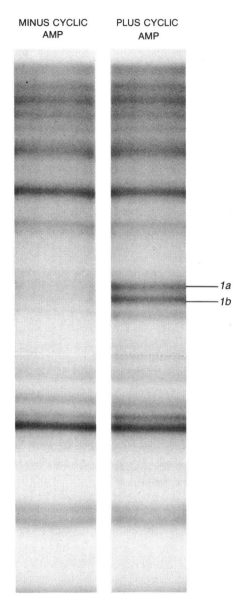

1a
1b

Figure 34 LONG-TERM EFFECTS of cyclic AMP on nerve-cell function are postulated to occur by the activation of a soluble protein kinase in the cytoplasm. Once activated this enzyme enters the cell nucleus, where it transfers a phosphate group from ATP to a nuclear regulatory protein closely associated with the DNA of inactive genes. Phosphorylation alters the shape or binding characteristics of the regulatory protein so that it dissociates from the DNA double helix, exposing the underlying stretch of DNA so that protein synthesis can occur. Proteins whose synthesis might be induced include neurotransmitter receptors, adenylate cyclases, structural proteins and enzymes involved in neurotransmitter synthesis or breakdown.

the suspension of red blood cells. Furthermore, by simultaneously measuring the state of phosphorylation of this protein and the movement of sodium ions into the cell in the presence of isoproterenol he has found that the time required for the membrane protein to reach half its maximum level of phosphorylation coincides closely with the time required for the flow of sodium ions across the membrane to reach half its maximum rate.

The results of these and other experiments conducted with a variety of systems demonstrate a close correlation between the movement of ions across cell membranes and the cyclic-AMP-dependent phosphorylation of specific membrane proteins. It should be pointed out, however, that correlation does not always mean causality. There is at present no direct proof that phosphorylation is a necessary event for the observed changes in permeability; both events could conceivably be secondary effects of some other process. The definitive proof of a causal connection between membrane-protein phosphorylation and permeability changes remains one of the major challenges for experimentation. We hope it will eventually be possible to dissect out the individual molecular components responsible for controlling ion permeability, put them into synthetic membranes and determine whether prior cyclic-AMP-dependent phosphorylation of one or more of these components will result in permeability changes similar to those observed in intact cells.

Because of the complex nature of cyclic-AMP-mediated processes, involving several biochemical steps, these processes are best suited to the regulation of synaptic events that are relatively long-lasting. This may be the reason the neuronal pathways that appear to make use of cyclic nucleotides often play a modulatory role in the nervous

Figure 33 SYNAPTIC MEMBRANES prepared from rat brain were incubated in a radioactive ATP solution in the presence or absence of added cyclic AMP, enabling molecules of protein kinase in the membrane to transfer a radioactive phosphate group from ATP to various substrate proteins. The phosphorylated proteins were removed from the membrane and separated by placing a mixture of them at the top of a column of gel-like polyacrylamide. High-voltage current caused the proteins to migrate downward and separate into thin bands. By placing the gels in a darkroom on X-ray film those bands that had incorporated radioactive phosphate were visible. Only two proteins (labeled *1a* and *1b*) were phosphorylated.

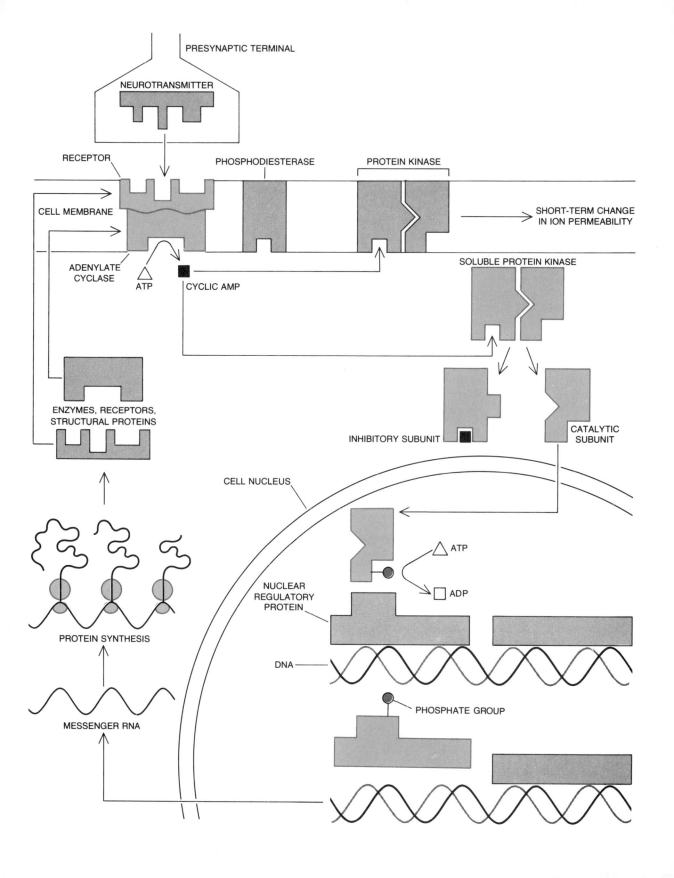

system, regulating activity rather than initiating it. For example, the cyclic AMP formed in the cerebellum by the activation of norepinephrine fibers in the locus coeruleus tones down the "spontaneous" firing rate of the Purkinje neurons. In ganglia of the sympathetic nervous system the dopamine synapses mediated by cyclic AMP adjust the level of activity at other synapses not mediated by cyclic AMP. Even in its role in movement disorders such as Parkinson's disease the cyclic AMP formed in the caudate nucleus by the activation of dopamine-sensitive adenylate cyclase appears to regulate movements only after they have been initiated by signals from other areas of the brain.

Observed changes in membrane excitability seen at cyclic-AMP-mediated synapses in the cerebellum and in the sympathetic ganglion may last for hundreds of milliseconds or longer—a long time on the scale of neural events. Recent investigations by Eric R. Kandel of Columbia University College of Physicians and Surgeons, working with a ganglion in a mollusk, and by Benjamin Libet of the University of California School of Medicine at San Francisco, working with a ganglion in the sympathetic nervous system of the rabbit, have demonstrated events of even greater duration that appear to be related to cyclic AMP, some of them lasting for hours. Observations such as these support the possibility that synaptic events mediated by cyclic nucleotides could be the basis for certain long-term changes in the central nervous system of man.

This notion has been supported by evidence indicating that the phosphorylation of protein mediated by cyclic AMP may influence events in the nucleus of the cell. A number of investigators, starting with Thomas A. Langan of the University of Colorado School of Medicine, have shown that histones, positively charged proteins that bind to the negatively charged phosphate backbone of the double helix of DNA, are susceptible to phosphorylation by a cyclic-AMP-dependent protein kinase. When histones are intimately associated with DNA, they appear to inhibit the expression of the DNA's information content by blocking access to the enzymes that effect the transcription of DNA to RNA. Phosphorylation by protein kinase makes the charge of the histones more negative, thereby reducing their ability to bind to DNA.

From a mechanistic point of view the linkage between adenylate cyclase and protein kinase supplies a ready-made system for the transformation of short-term synaptic events into longer-lived bio-

chemical changes. The cyclic AMP generated as a result of synaptic activity could conceivably activate a protein kinase, which would phosphorylate histone or some other nuclear regulatory protein and cause its removal from the DNA of inactive genes. The exposed genes would then be available for transcription into messenger RNA and ultimately translation into protein. Indeed, experiments in the laboratory of Erimino Costa at the National Institute of Mental Health suggest that cyclic AMP can induce the synthesis of tyrosine hydroxylase, an enzyme involved in the manufacture of dopamine and norepinephrine.

Thus the cyclic AMP system provides a mechanism by which the continued activation of a particular synapse could lead to the synthesis of new enzyme molecules or new receptor molecules, permanently altering the electrical properties of the receiving neuron. Whether such changes could constitute a molecular basis for information storage in the nervous system is hard to say, but it is certainly an attractive hypothesis. One can even speculate that the cyclic-AMP-dependent phosphorylation of synaptic-membrane proteins represents a type of short-term memory and that the phosphorylation of nuclear proteins and the synthesis of new protein molecules could represent a more permanent change—a long-term memory.

In sum, there exists in the brain a continuum of functional events that stretches from the brief to the very long-lived. At the short end of the scale are synaptic events, such as the contraction of voluntary muscle, that last for only a few milliseconds; at the long end are memories that can last for 50 years or more. On the basis of our present knowledge it seems possible that all but the very briefest of these events may involve cyclic-AMP-associated mechanisms.

Most of this discussion has emphasized the possible role of cyclic AMP in synapses and its importance in mediating the effects of many neurotransmitters and the actions of drugs that affect behavior. These areas have been a major focus of research on the role of cyclic nucleotides in the nervous system largely because of the conceptual and mechanistic analogies between the action of hormones and the transmission of nerve impulses. Mostly because of a comparative lack of evidence other roles for cyclic nucleotides in the nervous system have been somewhat underplayed. Considerable research over the past two or three years, both in our laboratory and elsewhere, suggests, however, that processes mediated by cyclic nucleotides are involved not only in the mechanism of changes in ion permeability induced by neurotransmitters but also in the regulation of a variety of other phenomena, including the activation of enzymes, the synthesis and release of neurotransmitters, intracellular movements, carbohydrate metabolism in the cere-

brum and possibly even processes of growth and development. We shall not elaborate on these recent advances, but we should like to emphasize their potential importance to an overall understanding of the functioning of the nervous system.

In particular, it may be useful to view the synaptic and nonsynaptic actions of cyclic AMP not so much in isolation but rather as part of an integrating sys-

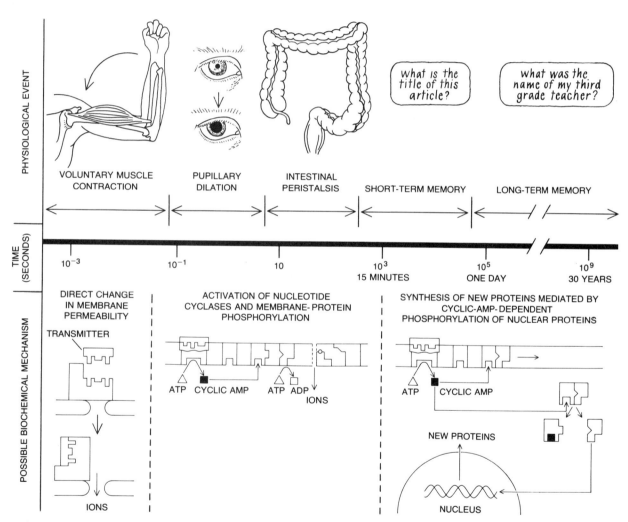

Figure 35 CONTINUUM OF SYNAPTIC EVENTS in the nervous system. At the short end of the spectrum are processes that are initiated in the span of a few milliseconds by the direct action of a neurotransmitter to open an ion channel in the membrane. Events lasting from hundreds of milliseconds to minutes appear to be mediated indirectly through the neurotransmitter-induced synthesis of cyclic

AMP, which initiates the phosphorylation of membrane proteins to produce a slow change in ion permeability. Events ranging from hours to years may involve the synthesis of new proteins directed by the cyclic-AMP-stimulated phosphorylation of proteins that regulate gene expression.

tem. It may be that enough synaptic stimulation not only raises cyclic AMP levels sufficiently to alter the permeability of membranes but also initiates a logical sequence of events mediated by cyclic nucleotides. This sequence might include a decrease or an increase in the synthesis of a neurotransmitter in response to synaptic stimulation, an initiation of intracellular movements in order to transport newly synthesized products, the activation of carbohydrate metabolism to supply the necessary cellular energy requirements, and direct effects on the genetic material in the cell nucleus that may lead to long-term alterations of behavior, such as memory.

POSTSCRIPT

Since 1977 the role of phosphoproteins in neuronal function has seen a true renaissance. An extraordinarily large number of phosphoproteins have been encountered in central and peripheral nervous systems. They are unquestionably related to the modulation of ionic channel activity and, indeed, may increase or decrease voltage- and ligand-activated channel conductances. In fact, one of the steps in the response to G protein activation is to effect phosphorylation. Equally impressive, most membrane receptors seem to be desensitized by protein phosphorylation. Phosphorylation regulates seven categories of neuronal proteins, enzymes involved in neurotransmitter biosynthesis, neurotransmitter receptors, ion channels, enzymes involved in cyclic nucleotide metabolism, autophosphorylated protein kinases, proteins involved in the regulation of transcription and translation and cytoskeletal proteins. In short, almost every aspect of neuronal activity seems to be under the control of phosphoproteins. (See the review by Greengard, 1987.)

Calcium in Synaptic Transmission

A current of calcium ions triggers the passage of signals from one nerve cell to another. The process is studied in a synapse (a neuronal junction) hundreds of times a synapse's usual size.

· · ·

Rodolfo R. Llinás

October, 1982

Synapses are the sites at which neurons, or nerve cells, communicate with one another. At an earlier stage in the life of an organism they are important in determining how the nervous system develops. (Synapses form at the tips of the fibers that sprout from the body of a neuron.) It seems certain that much of the brain's ability to regenerate after injury and much of an organism's ability to learn will ultimately be explained in terms of the function of synapses. Furthermore, it is becoming clear that most of the diseases of the brain and many psychiatric disorders result from a disruption of synaptic communication or are associated with such a disruption. The synapses is the weakest link in brain activity: it is the first part of a neuronal chain to be fatigued by a high level of message transmission, and it is the site of action for most of the drugs that affect the brain, including addictive substances as well as therapeutic ones from aspirin to barbiturates. For all these reasons a detailed understanding of every aspect of synaptic transmission is essential if we are to understand how the brain works and how the brain can malfunction.

Here I shall be concerned in particular with the aspect of transmission called depolarization-release coupling. In synaptic transmission one neuron (the presynaptic cell) releases a biologically active substance (a neurotransmitter), which evokes a response, either excitatory or inhibitory, in a second neuron (the postsynaptic cell). The release of the transmitter is in essence a process of secretion, a process shared by cells throughout the evolutionary sequence. In virtually every known instance secretion is accomplished by exocytosis, a mechanism in which vesicles, or membranous sacs, inside the cell fuse with the membrane that surrounds the cell. The fusion everts the contents of the vesicles into the extracellular environment.

A neuron evidently releases neurotransmitter in the same way. The release is known to be stimulated when the membrane of the presynaptic neuron at the synapse loses its electrical polarization. The step in synaptic transmission that concerns me here can be expressed, then, by a question: How does the depolarization of the membrane lead to the release of neurotransmitter, so that the neuron can act on the next cell in the neuronal chain? It turns out that the connection between the electrical activity of the cell and the release of neurotransmitter is not direct; an essential intermediary is the calcium ion.

When a neuron is at rest, there is an electric potential, or voltage difference, of some 70 millivolts between the inside of the cell and the outside. The voltage is negative inside, and so the cell membrane is said to have a polarization of −70 millivolts. When the membrane is depolarized, the voltage difference diminishes. Indeed, in the type of depolarization called the action potential a reverse potential develops with a value of from +10 to +30 millivolts. The reversal persists for only about a millisecond.

The precise mechanism by which depolarization arises is inconsequential as far as the subsequent release of neurotransmitter is concerned. In neurons such as sensory receptors that respond to stimuli (a burst of sound, a touch on the skin) impinging directly on the surface of the cell, the depolarization is caused by the energy of the stimulus itself. In such a neuron the depolarization can be a subtle change in potential that lasts for many seconds. In neurons in the brain the depolarization is generally caused by the signals each cell receives at the synapses it makes with other neurons. Here the depolarization is typically a rapid modulation in voltage that lasts for only a few milliseconds. If it is sufficiently great, it can induce the cell to generate its own action potential. In every case, however, the effect of a

wave of depolarization arriving at the membrane of the presynaptic terminal of a neuron is the same: it causes transmitter to be released.

Depolarization is nonetheless not sufficient in itself to cause the release of transmitter. In addition a supply of calcium ions must be present in the extracellular environment. Depolarization seems to be the means by which an inward current of calcium ions is induced to flow through the membrane of the presynaptic terminal. In this respect too synaptic transmission resembles other known secretory processes. In every secretory process in which the test has been made secretion is triggered by an increase in the concentration of calcium inside the secretory cell. The increase is the result of the entry of calcium from the external environment or of the release of calcium from internal stores. It seems likely that in neurons the entering calcium ions promote the fusion of special intracellular vesicles (synaptic vesicles) into the presynaptic membrane. The vesicles are stationed near the inner surface of the membrane at the site of transmitter release and are filled with the transmitter substance.

Among the difficulties that arise in attempts to advance our understanding beyond these basic points, one problem is implacable: synapses are small. So far the only measuring technique fast enough and precise enough to serve in the study of events in a functioning synapse is the recording of its electrical activity. Yet the diameter of a presynaptic terminal in most vertebrate and invertebrate species is typically from .1 micrometer to five mi-

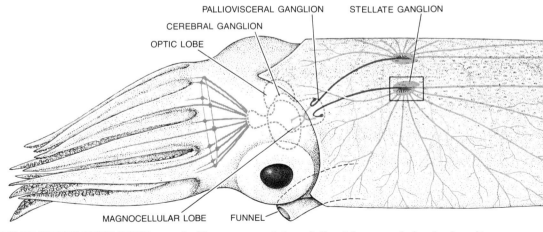

PALLIOVISCERAL GANGLION   STELLATE GANGLION
CEREBRAL GANGLION
OPTIC LOBE

MAGNOCELLULAR LOBE   FUNNEL

Figure 36 CHAIN OF GIANT NERVE CELLS on each side of the midline in the squid *Loligo pealii*, which includes a giant synapse. The first-order giant neuron (*green*) gathers sensory data and dispatches neural signals along its axon to the palliovisceral ganglion. The axon establishes synaptic contact with the second-order giant neuron (*red*). That

crometers. The microelectrode with which one can probe the synapse's electrical properties has a diameter of about .5 micrometer. Piercing the presynaptic terminal without damaging the synapse is quite difficult, and so is keeping the electrode in place as the experiment proceeds.

Fortunately for the experimenter some synapses are considerably larger than the average. They include certain synapses found in ganglia (clusters of neurons) in mollusks and crustaceans and the synapse between the neurons called Mauthner cells in the brain stem of fishes and some amphibians. The Mauthner cells govern the movement of the tail. Among large synapses, however, the most notable example is a giant synapse of the squid. It is some 700 micrometers long. Because of its size and accessibility it has yielded most of what is now known directly about the relation of depolarization to the release of neurotransmitter.

The presence of a giant synapse in the squid was first reported in 1935 by J. Z. Young of the Marine Biological Association of the United Kingdom at Plymouth. The synapse was included in his description of a chain of giant nerve cells in the squid (see Figure 36); the chain consists of three axons, or nerve fibers, and the neuronal cell bodies from which they arise. The axons' diameters are so great that some of them had been mistaken for blood vessels; Young identified them as nervous tissue on the basis of their ability to conduct an action potential. The chains on each side of the

squid's body are now known to govern the animal's flight response and capture of prey.

The first nerve cell in the chain is called the first-order giant neuron. It is in the magnocellular lobe, an assemblage of neurons in what amounts to the animal's brain. Its cell body is some 150 micrometers in diameter, which makes it many times larger than the largest nerve cells in the human brain. With its extensive set of dendrites (tubular extensions of the cell body) it is 800 micrometers long. By means of these dendrites it gathers signals that originate in such places as the eyes, the vestibular organs and the tentacles. It is in effect a single-cell computer that assesses danger to the animal. The results of its calculations are transmitted along the membrane of its axon. As if to ensure the synchrony of such signals, the axons of the first-order giant neurons on each side of the body fuse for a short distance at the midline.

The second cell in the chain, the second-order giant neuron, is in the palliovisceral ganglion behind the magnocellular lobe. The second-order cell is 100 micrometers in diameter. Its axon curves through the ganglion on a trajectory that directs it toward the squid's mantle. Along the curve it comes in contact with the axon of the first-order giant cell, which establishes a synapse with it. Then the second-order axon continues on to the center of the stellate ganglion (see Figures 36 and 37), on the inner surface of the mantle. There it broadens and divides into a set of from eight to 10 terminal branches that look like fingers radiating

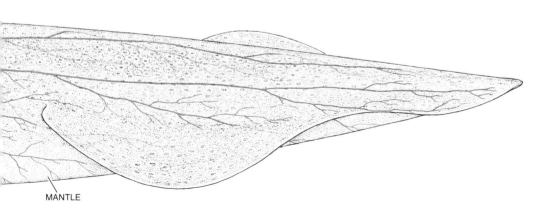

MANTLE

fiber proceeds to the stellate ganglion and synaptically contacts a set of third-order axons (*blue*) that trigger the mantle's contraction. The contraction sends water jetting out of the animal's funnel, propelling it from danger. The stellate ganglion enclosed by a rectangle is enlarged in Figure 37.

from the palm of a hand. The branches vary in size: the thinnest are 25 micrometers in diameter and the thickest are twice as big.

The third cell in the chain is actually a set of hundreds of cells, each of which is about 50 micrometers in diameter. The cells are organized into from eight to 10 sets, and in each set all the axons fuse to form a single giant axon. Hence the stellate ganglion gives rise to from eight to 10 giant axons. The thinnest of them is about 50 micrometers in diameter; it receives signals through a synapse with the thinnest of the terminal branches of the second-order axon, then it widens somewhat and proceeds away from the stellate ganglion to innervate muscle tissue in the mantle near the ganglion. The thickest of the third-order axons is about 200 micrometers in diameter; it receives signals through a synapse with the thickest of the terminal branches of the second-order axon, then it widens to a diameter of about 500 micrometers and extends to innervate muscle tissue in the most distant part of the mantle. The other third-order axons have intermediate destinations.

The rudiments of how this network functions can be inferred from its structure. When stimuli reaching the first-order neuron exceed some threshold that signifies alarm, the cell activates the second-order axon, which in turn produces a synchronous excitation in all the third-order axons. The speed with which a wave of depolarization propagates along a nerve fiber depends on the diameter of the fiber; since the longest of the third-order axons are also the thickest, the synchronization of the signals is preserved and all the muscles of the mantle contract simultaneously. The contraction forces the water in the mantle out through the funnel near the head of the animal. Thus the squid can escape from danger by jet propulsion.

The giant synapse we have studied is the one between the second-order axon and the largest third-order axon. When the synapse is examined in detail, it is found that the membrane of the presynaptic terminal (the second-order axon) is smooth. In contrast, the membrane of the postsynaptic terminal (the third-order axon) has multiple branchings that divide repeatedly and end as a net of thorn-shaped

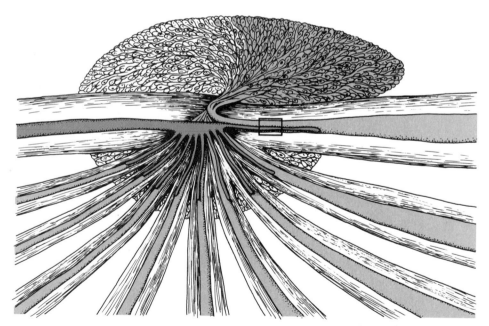

Figure 37 IN THE STELLATE GANGLION the second-order axon (*red*) branches into a series of presynaptic terminals. Each makes synaptic contact with a third-order axon (*blue*), which arises from the fusion of the axons emitted by several hundred neurons in the ganglion known as the giant fiber lobe. The largest third-order axon, shown leaving the ganglion to the right at the center of a bundle of smaller axons, forms the postsynaptic part of the giant synapse. The part of the synapse enclosed by the rectangle is enlarged in Figure 38.

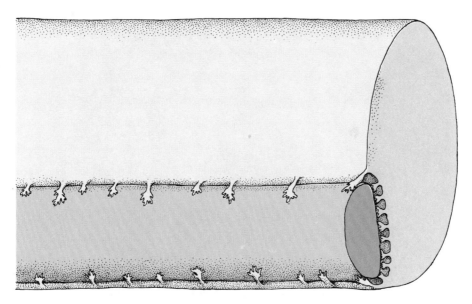

Figure 38 GIANT SYNAPSE is made up of two apposed membranes. The postsynaptic membrane of the third-order axon has some 5,000 spiny extensions. They face the presynaptic membrane.

extensions. In the giant synapse as many as 5,000 such extensions face the presynaptic membrane (see Figure 38). This structure is unusual. In a typical synapse the postsynaptic terminal is smooth, whereas the presynaptic terminal consists of protuberances at the end of an axon that are called synaptic boutons (from the French word for button).

Nevertheless, a microscopic examination of the places in the giant synapse where the presynaptic membrane abuts a postsynaptic thorn shows morphology quite typical of a synapse. Inside the presynaptic terminal at such places there are synaptic vesicles and two other intracellular structures that are notably abundant at synapses: mitochondria, the organelles that make energy available to the cell, and subcysternal systems, which consist of folds of intracellular membrane. (The function of the latter is not known.) In the same areas the postsynaptic thorn has a thickened membrane, which is recognized in the typical synapse to be the site where receptors are found. The receptors are molecules embedded in the postsynaptic membrane that react with arriving molecules of neurotransmitter.

It was in the giant synapse of the squid that it was first demonstrated directly that the transmission of a neural signal across the synapse requires the release of a transmitter substance. This intermediate chemical step (first proposed in the course of research on the union between nerve and muscle) was established in the 1950's and the early 1960's through a number of studies by Theodore H. Bullock, Susumu Hagiwara, Ichiji Tasaki, Noriko and Akira Takeuchi, Ricardo Miledi and C. R. Slater. The studies capitalized on the size of the giant synapse: the workers were able to position the tip of a microelectrode in the presynaptic terminal and the tip of a second microelectrode in the postsynaptic axon so that the voltage across the membrane of each terminal could be recorded simultaneously. In addition the workers could vary the concentration of ions or drugs in the solution in which they had isolated the synapse (along with a few centimeters of the second-order and third-order axons). Thus they could study the role of the ions and the action of the drugs.

It emerged from the various studies that when an action potential propagating along the second-order axon reaches the presynaptic terminal, it causes a depolarization of the postsynaptic axon after a delay of about a millisecond. On the other hand, an action potential at the postsynaptic terminal (induced by electrical stimulation of the third-order axon) has no effect on the presynaptic terminal. It further emerged that the degree of postsynaptic de-

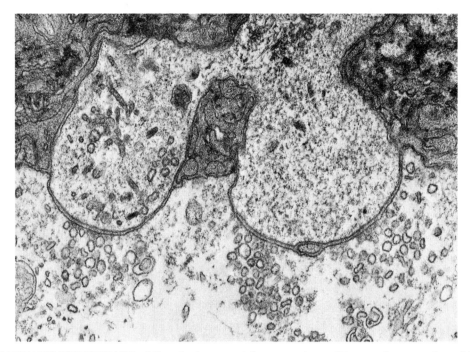

Figure 39 ELECTRON MICROGRAPH of the giant synapse. The presynaptic terminal of the synapse is at the bottom, abutted by two bulbous protrusions arising from a single spiny extension of the postsynaptic axon. Inside the presynaptic terminal at the places of abutment are accumulations of synaptic vesicles, which are thought to contain a neurotransmitter: a substance released by the presynaptic terminal that acts on the membrane of the postsynaptic terminal. (Micrograph by D. W. Pumplin at the University of Maryland Baltimore School of Medicine and T. S. Reese at the National Institute of Neurological and Communicative Disorders and Stroke.)

polarization increases with the amplitude and the duration of the presynaptic action potential. Yet the presynaptic action potential becomes incapable of causing postsynaptic depolarization if all the calcium is removed from the solution in which the synapse is bathed. The combination of all these findings (showing, among other things, synaptic delay and unidirectionality) was strong evidence that signals are not transmitted electrically across the giant synapse. They are carried by a chemical messenger.

In 1966 Bernard Katz and Miledi, working at the Zoological Station in Naples, and two groups working at the Marine Biological Laboratory in Woods Hole, Mass., one group consisting of Kiyoshi Kusano, D. R. Livengood and Robert Werman and the other of James R. Bloedel, Peter W. Gage, David M. J. Quastel and me, made a further discovery. Signal transmission across the giant synapse does not require the arrival of a presynaptic action potential. It requires only that the presynaptic terminal be depolarized, which can be accomplished not only by an action potential but also by passing an electric current into the terminal through a microelectrode that impales it. The discovery was significant because it separated the mechanism of electrical excitability responsible for the action potential from the mechanism responsible for the release of transmitter from the presynaptic terminal.

The amount of transmitter released by the presynaptic terminal under artificial stimulation turned out to depend in a curious way on the degree of presynaptic depolarization. A slight depolarization of the presynaptic membrane causes a small postsynaptic depolarization; hence one infers that a relatively small amount of transmitter is released from the presynaptic terminal. A larger presynaptic depolarization leads to a larger response, but only up to a point: the response decreases if the presynaptic depolarization is greater than 60 millivolts with respect to its resting value of −70 millivolts, or in other words if the presynaptic potential attains a value more positive than −10 millivolts. If the presynaptic depolarization is great enough, so that the presynaptic potential becomes greater than +60 millivolts, the postsynaptic response can actually disappear. Even then, however, brief synaptic transmission is detected at the end of the experimental pulse as the presynaptic potential returns to its resting value.

These observations were interpreted in terms of the effect of depolarization on the flow of calcium ions. When the neuron is in its resting state, the membrane is impermeable to calcium ions, which have a much higher concentration outside the cell than inside. Depolarization evidently opens channels in the membrane that allow calcium ions to pass; as a result the ions flow inward, propelled by

the electromotive force arising from what remains of the electric potential across the membrane as well as the lesser concentration of calcium inside the terminal. If the depolarization is sufficiently strong, however, the influx of ions is opposed by electrical forces. The calcium ion carries two positive electric charges, and when the interior of the cell becomes electrically positive, the ions are repelled. Thus even though the membrane channels are opened by the depolarization, the calcium ions cannot enter the cell and neurotransmitter is not released. The degree of presynaptic depolarization at which synaptic transmission is abolished was named the suppression potential, and the postsynaptic response at the end of a pulse was named the off postsynaptic potential.

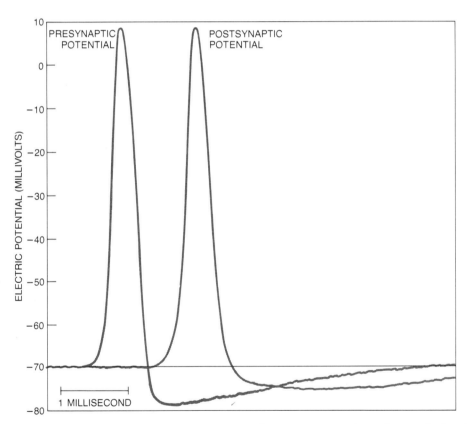

Figure 40 NORMAL ELECTRICAL ACTIVITY at the giant synapse resembles the activity at synapses in all vertebrate and invertebrate animals. When the electric potential across the membrane of the presynaptic terminal is altered from its resting value of −70 millivolts by a voltage spike called an action potential, the presynaptic terminal releases neurotransmitter whose arrival at the postsynaptic terminal alters the permeability of the postsynaptic membrane to ions. The resulting ionic current through the membrane stimulates the postsynaptic terminal to develop a voltage spike.

The early results of the study of the giant synapse lent support, then, to the hypothesis, first proposed by Katz, that calcium triggers the release of neurotransmitter. Still, the calcium hypothesis came of age only when the results of three further lines of investigation became known in the late 1960's and early 1970's.

First, Katz and Miledi demonstrated that calcium ions are capable of generating action potentials, but only at the presynaptic terminal, and that these action potentials are accompanied by the release of transmitter. In particular they demonstrated that if the ability of the presynaptic membrane to pass sodium and potassium ions is blocked by drugs, action potentials can nonetheless be detected along with a subsequent postsynaptic depolarization. What modulates the voltage across the membrane of a neuron as an action potential propagates is the redistribution of ions and hence of electric charge between the interior of the cell and the extracellular environment. Sodium ions flow in; then potassium ions flow out. The action potentials Katz and Miledi detected must have depended entirely on the passage of calcium ions. From their results they inferred that the presynaptic membrane has calcium channels. The action potentials were abolished when calcium was removed from the bathing solution.

Second, Miledi did a much simpler experiment. He showed that in the absence of extracellular calcium the mere injection of calcium ions into the presynaptic terminal causes a postsynaptic depolarization. Therefore the injected calcium must have caused transmitter to be released.

The third line of work was done by John R. Blinks, Charles Nicholson and me. We showed that if the presynaptic terminal is filled with aequorin, a protein that emits light when it is exposed to calcium, light can be detected in the presynaptic terminal during normal synaptic transmission. It follows that the concentration of calcium in the terminal increases at such times. A further experiment by Nicholson and me showed that the light signals synaptic events quite faithfully. For example, when we applied a suppression potential to the presynaptic terminal, we failed to detect light during the depolarizing pulse. We did detect light when we stopped the pulse and the postsynaptic terminal responded with an off potential. This demonstrated that the suppression of transmission is indeed due specifically to a suppression of the entry of calcium ions.

Beyond all doubt, then, calcium is the agent that triggers synaptic transmission. Two points remained to be clarified: the relation between depolarization and the entry of calcium and the subsequent relation between the entry of calcium and the release of transmitter. With this in mind my colleagues and I decided to make a change in our experimental technique. In essence we had been using a current clamp: we had injected into the presynaptic terminal a constant electric current and measured the resulting presynaptic depolarization (the changing voltage across the membrane of the terminal). The membrane has the electrical properties of resistance and capacitance, that is, it resists the flow of electric current and also stores electric charge, causing a delay in its response to a current pulse. In general, therefore, the procedure of current clamping resembles the charging of a capacitor in parallel with a resistor and the measurement of the voltage across the pair.

The difficulty with the current-clamping method is that the electrical properties of the membrane of a neuron are more complex than those of a capacitor in parallel with a resistor. Specifically, the changing voltage across the membrane can open channels that allow various kinds of ions (including calcium ions) to enter and leave the neuron. In short, the membrane's conductivity to ions is voltage-dependent. The movements of ions (which constitute an electric current) cause further changes in the voltage, which cause still further changes in the membrane, and so on. The most extreme result of this membrane self-modulation is an action potential. Learning the properties of the membrane when it is actively changing its voltage and no longer responding passively to experimental manipulation is problematic. Yet the active properties of the membrane are central to a nerve cell's functioning.

We determined, therefore, to end our work with current-clamping and take the opposite tack: we would employ the voltage-clamp technique that Kenneth S. Cole had devised at the Marine Biological Laboratory. A. L. Hodgkin and A. F. Huxley of the University of Cambridge had employed the technique to elucidate (in the third-order giant axon of the squid) the electrical events underlying the action potential. In the voltage-clamp technique a burst of current drives the membrane of a neuron very rapidly to a given level of depolarization. The level is then kept constant ("clamped") in spite of the movement of ions through channels that have opened in the membrane. The clamping is accom-

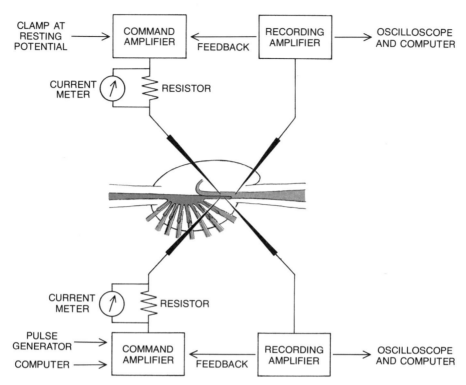

Figure 41 VOLTAGE-CLAMP CIRCUITRY imposes a predetermined pattern of voltage on the presynaptic or postsynaptic terminal or both of them. One microelectrode monitors the voltage across the membrane of the presynaptic terminal. Its measurements serve as feedback for a second microelectrode, which injects current into the terminal. Instruments monitor the amount of current injected to give the terminal a "clamped" voltage, set by a pulse generator or a computer. A similar method clamps the postsynaptic terminal at its resting potential.

plished by an electronic feedback circuit that varies the continuing injection of current.

The voltage-clamp technique has two advantages. First, the amount of current injected when the clamp is in effect must exactly balance the current of ions; hence the metering of the applied current constitutes a measurement of the ionic current. It is a measurement that cannot otherwise be made, since the microelectrodes record only voltages. Second, the step in voltage that marks the onset of the clamping is much faster than the changes it induces in the structure of the membrane. This means the clamp circuitry charges the membrane's capacitance well before ionic currents have started to flow through membrane channels. It follows that the ionic currents can be distinguished from the injected current that merely gets stored in the terminal; therefore we could hope in our further work with the giant synapse to study the full time course of changes in the presynaptic membrane's conductivity (or equivalently the opening and closing of channels and the passage of ions through them) for a given steady level of depolarization. Indeed, we could hope to derive from measurements of the current of calcium ions at various levels of clamped depolarization a mathematical model of the presynaptic calcium conductance, that is, a mathematical expression that would suggest how the membrane's calcium channels change in response to a changing pattern of voltage.

During the summers of 1975 through 1978 Kerry Walton and I did a series of voltage-clamp experiments at the Marine Biological Laboratory (see Figure 42). We blocked the conductance of the presynaptic membrane to sodium and potassium, so that our measurements would represent only the flow of calcium ions. We found to our delight that the calcium current was readily measured. It turns out that the membrane's conductivity to calcium depends in a complex way on the level of clamped depolarization.

Consider the time course of the current. In response to a small step of depolarizing voltage the calcium current increases quite slowly: it reaches a plateau only after several milliseconds. In response to a larger voltage step it attains its plateau value in a fraction of a millisecond. Consider also the amplitude of the plateau. Almost no calcium current is detected unless the voltage step is at least 15 millivolts. For a larger step the plateau amplitude is

markedly greater. For a step of 60 millivolts (which gives the terminal membrane a clamped potential of −10 millivolts) the amplitude is maximal. For still larger steps the amplitude decreases, a result that Katz and Miledi's discovery of the suppression potential would lead one to expect. For clamp potentials greater than +60 millivolts the current is again quite small.

At the end of an episode of clamping the presynaptic potential falls from its clamped value back to the resting value of −70 millivolts. The return to resting potential (which can be accomplished

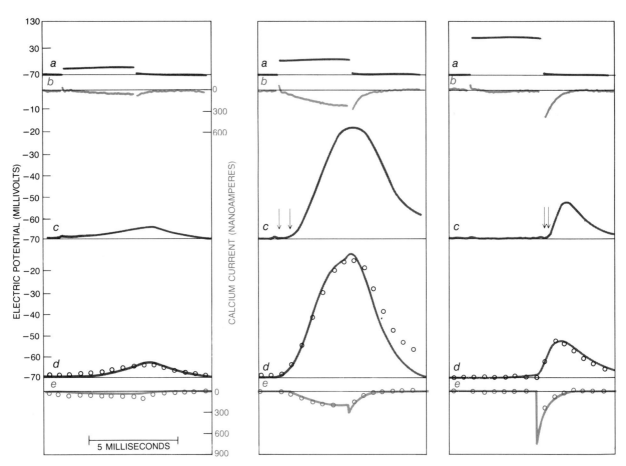

Figure 42 VOLTAGE-CLAMP EXPERIMENTS subjected the presynaptic terminal of the giant synapse to an artificial "step" in voltage (a), of 30 (*left graph*), 52 (*middle*) and 130 millivolts (*right*). The current across the membrane (b) represented the flow of calcium ions. The calcium influx into the presynaptic terminal causes neurotransmitter to be released, as indicated by the presence of a potential in the postsynaptic terminal (c). Arrows indicate the "synaptic delay." The data collected in the experiments yield a model of synaptic transmissions. At the bottom the postsynaptic potential (d) and the presynaptic calcium current (e) resulting from the model are compared with the experimental data (*dots*).

quickly by the voltage-clamp circuitry) is accompanied by a second and distinctive flow of calcium ions into the presynaptic terminal. It is called the tail current, and it has been observed for ions other than calcium. It has no delay: it starts as soon as the voltage step ends.

The tail current can be explained as follows. Throughout the voltage step the calcium channels in the presynaptic membrane are open, and at the end of the step they close. The closing of the channels, however, is slower than the return of the potential to its resting value. The channels therefore remain open briefly after the potential has decayed, at a time when the electromotive force again is favorable for the entry of calcium ions.

Doubtless the tail current is responsible for the release of transmitter that causes the off postsynaptic response. It is remarkable, then, that the off response begins a mere .2 millisecond after the tail current starts to flow. It is all the more remarkable because the normal postsynaptic response to the arrival of an action potential at the presynaptic terminal is delayed by as much as a millisecond. One must conclude that a large part of the synaptic delay is due to the time required for the calcium channels to open when the presynaptic membrane is first depolarized. The subsequent events in synaptic transmission must be fast indeed. In particular, once calcium ions have entered the presynaptic terminal they must act quite rapidly to get transmitter released.

The next goal of our work was to devise from our data a mathematical description relating the calcium current to any given pattern of voltage. To this end we began a collaboration with Izchak Z. Steinberg of the Weizmann Institute of Science in Israel. The heart of such a mathematical model is a description of how the calcium channels in the membrane respond to depolarization. The hypotheses with which Steinberg, Walton and I began were similar to those proposed by Hodgkin and Huxley for sodium and potassium channels. We assumed that a driving force arises from the difference between the concentration of calcium ions inside the presynaptic terminal and the concentration outside it. We further assumed that an increase in the presynaptic membrane's conductivity to calcium ions can be triggered by voltage-dependent changes in the structure of calcium channels that cause them to open. One of the simplest possibilities is that each channel consists of a certain number of subunits

and that each subunit has two possible states, s and s'. Probably each state corresponds to a different shape. If all the subunits in a channel are in the state s' (the activated state), the channel is open; otherwise it is closed. The probability that a subunit will enter state s' is determined by the voltage across the membrane; the greater the extent of depolarization is, the more likely the subunit is to be activated. One further assumption is that the subunits do not interact with one another but that each subunit changes its shape independently.

From these assumptions (together with the laws of thermodynamics) it is possible to construct a family of equations expressing the time course of the calcium current in response to a clamped presynaptic voltage. The current is proportional to the rate at which ions flow through an open gate multiplied by the fraction of the gates that are open. Each equation incorporates a different assumption about the number of subunits per gate. In the equation that best matches the time course and voltage-dependence of the calcium current we had measured in our voltage-clamp experiments the number of subunits is five.

One hypothetical configuration for the channel (a configuration offered in the absence of any direct evidence) is a set of five identical proteins, each one spanning the thickness of the presynaptic membrane; the five protein molecules might be arranged in the form of a rosette. When all the proteins have the shape s', they circumscribe a channel that allows the entry of calcium ions. Recently, however, the study of individual calcium channels by several investigators has suggested an alternative configuration in which each channel is circumscribed by a helix of proteins.

The voltage-clamp experiments show that the calcium current saturates, or attains a maximum value. Hence each channel must be able to pass only a certain number of calcium ions per unit of time regardless of the driving force. To explain the saturation we assume that each channel has an energy barrier. Perhaps a part of each protein molecule juts slightly into the channel and has a positive electric charge. Because the charge would tend to repel an entering calcium ion the driving force would have to "push" ions through the channel and their rate of flow would have an upper limit. The voltage-clamp experiments also show that the falloff in calcium current at the end of a voltage step is simply an exponential decrease and not the more gradual falloff that would indicate a complex sequence of

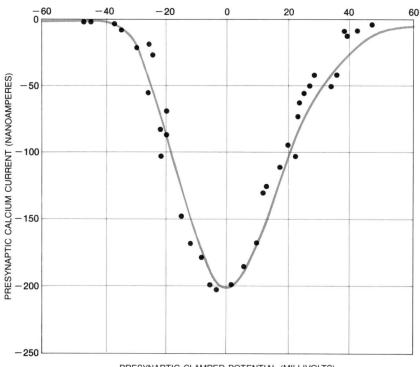

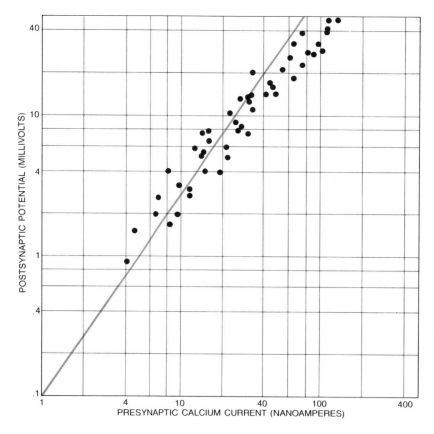

Figure 43 RESULTS OF VOLT-AGE-CLAMP EXPERIMENTS.
The relation between the clamped value of the presynaptic voltage and the plateau level of the calcium current that flows into the presynaptic terminal (*top graph*) is nonlinear: the current has its maximum for a clamped voltage of about −10 millivolts, and it is negligible for clamping above about 60 millivolts. The relation between the calcium current and the postsynaptic response (*bottom graph*) has a slope between one and two. Both axes in the bottom graph are logarithmic.

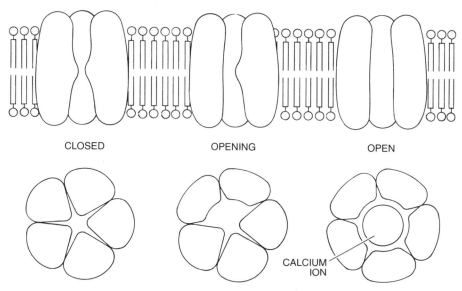

CLOSED   OPENING   OPEN

CALCIUM
ION

Figure 44 CALCIUM CHANNELS in the membrane of the presynaptic terminal must open in response to a change in voltage in order for the calcium current to flow. The model of synaptic transmission devised by the author and colleagues may hypothetically be represented by a rosette consisting of five proteins each of which extends through the membrane. The voltage must change the shape of all five proteins before calcium ions can enter.

events. This finding fits the hypothesis that a change in the shape of only one subunit in an open channel suffices to close it.

With a mathematical model for the response of the calcium channels to a given clamped level of voltage we could calculate the response of the channels to an arriving action potential. We approximated the action potential by a series of incremental changes in voltage and then we employed the model to predict the calcium current that would result from the succession of increments. We do not know the number of calcium channels in the presynaptic membrane, nor do we know the conductivity of an individual channel, and so the model's results could suggest not the actual magnitude of the calcium current but only its time course and its relative magnitude. Nevertheless, it appeared from the results that the calcium current starts to flow at the end of the action potential as the presynaptic voltage returns to its resting level.

Our third goal was to relate the presynaptic inflow of calcium to the release of neurotransmitter. Since the delay between the two events is only some .2 millisecond, we hypothesized that the calcium enters the presynaptic terminal quite near

the site where transmitter is released. We further supposed the latter site would be marked in electron micrographs by the presence of synaptic vesicles.

Electron microscopy of the giant synapse does indeed show "active zones." They are characterized by a gathering of vesicles in the presynaptic terminal and a thickening in the membrane of the postsynaptic terminal. Scanning electron micrographs made by the freeze-fracture method reveal additional structure. In the freeze-fracture technique a second of tissue including the giant synapse is frozen and then cracked. The tissue tends to cleave down the middle of either the presynaptic membrane or the postsynaptic one. Under the electron microscope the freeze-fracture specimens show that the presynaptic membrane at an active zone has embedded in it as many as 1,500 small particles. We hypothesize (with other investigators) that they are the sites of calcium entry.

In order to incorporate into our model the relation of calcium entry to transmitter release we made some further assumptions. They are again the simplest possibilities. In the presynaptic terminal we assume that calcium binds to a molecule we call the fusion-promoting factor. In response to the binding a certain part of the factor molecule enters an active state by way of a first-order kinetic reaction (a reaction whose overall rate depends only on the concentration of a single reactant, in this case the fusion-promoting factor itself).

The activated fusion-promoting factor causes synaptic vesicles to fuse with the presynaptic membrane so that they release their content of neurotransmitter. The rate of the reaction depends only on the concentration of the activated factor. Then the activated factor returns to an inactive state. Meanwhile the neurotransmitter molecules are opening channels in the postsynaptic membrane so

that ionic currents flow and the membrane becomes depolarized. The model resulting from these assumptions proved capable of reproducing the postsynaptic responses we had measured in the voltage-clamp experiments, including the postsynaptic off potential at the end of a presynaptic depolarization exceeding the suppression potential.

Thus far our voltage-clamp studies had yielded a set of experimental results amenable to a mathematical description of the presynaptic calcium current and its relation to the amplitude of the postsynaptic potential. Ultimately, however, the model had to be

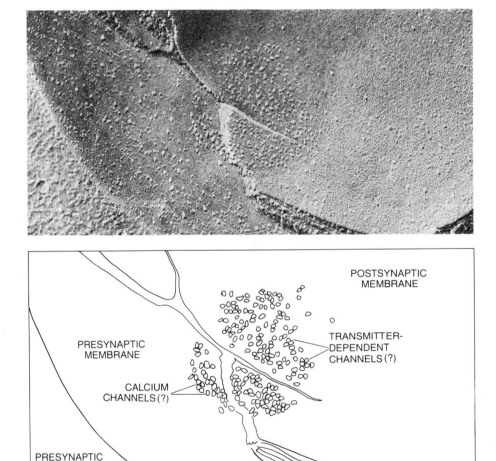

Figure 45 SMALL PARTICLES in the membrane of the presynaptic terminal may be the calcium channels. Particles in the postsynaptic membrane may be channels that open in response to the arrival of transmitter molecules. The tissue shown was frozen, then cracked, which charac- teristically splits a neuronal membrane down the middle (that is, between its lipid layers). Each particle is thus embedded in the membrane. (Micrograph by D. W. Pumplin and T. S. Reese.)

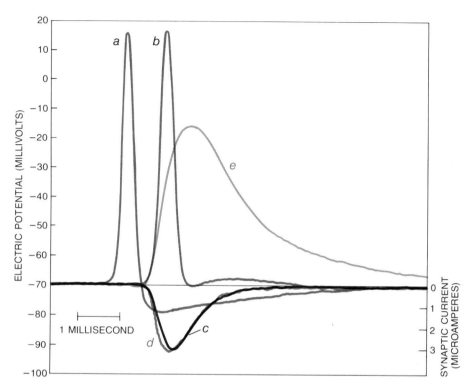

Figure 46 NATURAL ACTION POTENTIAL (*a*) **is recorded in the presynaptic terminal and produces a postsynaptic action potential** (*b*). **When the postsynaptic terminal is voltage-clamped at resting potential, the amount of current the clamp injects** (*c*) **is equal in time course and magnitude to the synaptic current through the postsynaptic membrane. Following blockage of the action potential** by drugs, the presynaptic voltage-clamp circuit can recreate an artificial action potential from computer memory. The resulting synaptic current (*d*) has the same latency, amplitude and time course as in natural events. If the postsynaptic terminal is unclamped but drugs remain, the terminal responds to the artificial action potential with a prolonged change in voltage (*e*).

tested against actual measurements of the calcium current during the course of an action potential. In 1979 and 1980 the test was attempted. In a series of experiments done by Mutsuyuki Sugimori, Sanford M. Simon and me at the Marine Biological Laboratory a presynaptic action potential and the resulting postsynaptic action potential were recorded simultaneously in the giant synapse. The recorded changes in membrane potential were stored in the memory of a digital computer. We then employed the recorded signals in experiments of a new kind.

As in the earlier voltage-clamp experiments the voltage-dependent conductance of the membranes for sodium and potassium was blocked chemically, leaving the presynaptic membrane with only its voltage-dependent conductance for calcium and leaving the postsynaptic membrane with only the ionic channels that are opened by the arrival of transmitter molecules. The new experiments differed in that we no longer clamped the presynaptic terminal at a constant level of depolarization. Instead the amplifier and the microelectrode that inject current into the presynaptic terminal were driven by the presynaptic voltage spike we had recorded earlier. In this way we artificially imposed on the terminal the voltage pattern of an action potential even though the normal basis of the action potential (the inward flow of sodium ions and the outward flow of potassium ions) was absent. The postsynaptic response to the artificial action potential was virtually identical with the response to the natural voltage spike; hence the artificial potential caused the release of transmitter from the presynaptic terminal with an identical amplitude and delay.

We felt justified, therefore, in thinking that fur-

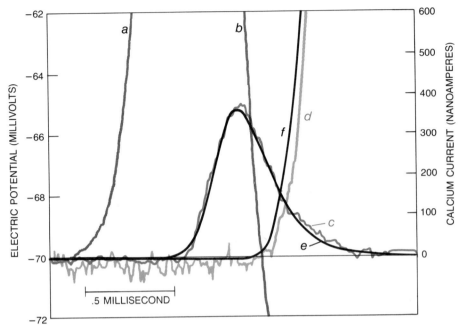

Figure 47 ROLE OF CALCIUM in synaptic transmission determined by artificial action potential. The artificial voltage spike is applied while sodium and potassium are blocked. Only the upshoot (*a*) and fall (*b*) of the artificial spike are visible. During its falling phase the presynaptic spike opens calcium channels and calcium current (*c*) flows into the preterminal fiber, triggering transmitter release. The postsynaptic response begins soon after (*d*). Also shown are the calcium current (*e*) and the postsynaptic response (*f*) predicted by the model.

ther measurements made when ionic conduction was suppressed and the presynaptic terminal was stimulated by an artificial action potential would be a valid representation of natural events. Accordingly, we monitored the amount of current the voltage-clamp circuitry injected into the presynaptic terminal to make the artificial spike. Since sodium and potassium currents were being blocked, the injected current had two components. Part of it depolarized the membrane and thereby made up for the absence of the sodium and potassium currents; the rest exactly counterbalanced the calcium current that was flowing unblocked through the membrane. Next we chemically blocked the calcium current and repeated the experiment. The difference between the two results is the calcium current alone. It compares closely with the calcium current predicted by our model.

Quite recently our results have been confirmed by the work of Steven J. Smith, Milton P. Charlton and Robert S. Zucker at the Marine Biological Laboratory and that of Miledi and Parker in Naples. The work employed a dye that changes color in the presence of calcium. The dye is injected into the presynaptic terminal of the giant synapse. Its change in color there suggests a time course for the calcium current much like the one we measured by voltage-clamping.

Many prospects are now before us. For some years I have been tantalized by the possibility that synaptic transmission is a modified form of neuronal growth. For one thing, the concentration of calcium in developing neural tissue seems to control the rate at which a growth cone, which is the growing tip of an axon, adds new cell membrane to its surface. Then too the membrane of a growth cone has a voltage-dependent conductance for calcium ions.

Perhaps the synaptic terminal can be regarded as a modified growth cone in which growth has been subdued, so that there is no longer any permanent increase in the area of the membrane. In an embryonic neuron vesicles in a growth cone might fuse with the growth-cone membrane to increase the extent of the membrane and give it newly minted proteins. Later in the life of the organism the vesicles in the presynaptic terminal that arises from the growth cone would fuse with the membrane of the terminal, evert their content of neurotransmitter and get taken back into the terminal. (Such recycling was proposed some years ago by John E. Heuser and Thomas S. Reese.) The mechanism that serves growth and plasticity in the developing nervous system would then come to serve neuronal signaling. The understanding of the molecular processes underlying this sequence of events holds the highest promise in the search for the ways of the brain.

POSTSCRIPT

We still do not understand exactly how cells can release the chemical transmitter substances that allow them to interact with other neurons. Since that is a most fundamental step in the functioning of the brain, our lack of comprehension is both frustrating and exhilarating, as this field of research promises to become quite "hot." There is the feeling that we are about to see the missing link between the operation of a synapse as described and the cell and molecular biology that makes it all happen. While the presynaptic calcium conductance is well understood, its role in triggering transmitter release remains obscure. One set of findings relates to a specific protein, Synapsin I, first identified by Paul Greengard. This protein, when injected into the presynaptic terminal in its dephosphorylated form, blocked transmitter release. It did so, most probably, by adhering to synaptic vesicles and forming a molecular cage that prevents the vesicles from fusing with the plasmamembrane. However, when phosphorylated Synapsin I was injected into the terminal, no modification of transmitter release was observed. Moreover, transmitter release was increased up to seven times when CAMkinase II, which phosphorylates Synapsin I, was presynaptically injected (Llinás et al., 1985). Dephosphoro-Synapsin I was directly related to changes in transmitter release by labeling it with Texas Red. The flow of Synapsin I was monitored and the decrease in transmitter release was found to follow closely its degree of invasions of the preterminal fiber, indicating that Synapsin I operates locally at the site of release.

Another area that has received much attention relates to the refinement of the "calcium hypothesis" of transmitter release. It has been proposed that bulk intracellular calcium concentration is not the operant variable in release, but rather the calcium concentration in the immediate vicinity of the intracellular opening of calcium channels. The issue is one of microcompartmentalization of the intracellular calcium domain (Simon el al., 1984; Chad and Eckert, 1984; Simon and Llinás, 1985 and Zucker and Fogelson, 1986). An excellent review of calcium in transmitter release was published in 1987 by Augustine, Charlton and Smith.

Small Systems of Neurons

Such systems are the elementary units of mental function. Studies of simple animals such as the large snail Aplysia *show that small systems of neurons are capable of forms of learning and memory.*

• • •

Eric R. Kandel

September, 1979

Many neurobiologists believe that the unique character of individual human beings, their disposition to feel, think, learn and remember, will ultimately be shown to reside in the precise patterns of synaptic interconnections between the neurons of the brain. Since it is difficult to examine patterns of interconnections in the human brain, a major concern of neurobiology has been to develop animal models that are useful for studying how interacting systems of neurons give rise to behavior. Networks of neurons that mediate complete behavioral acts allow one to explore a hierarchy of interrelated questions: To what degree do the properties of different neurons vary? What determines the patterns of interconnections between neurons? How do different patterns of interconnections generate different forms of behavior? Can the interconnected neurons that control a certain kind of behavior be modified by learning? If they can, what are the mechanisms whereby memory is stored?

Among the many functions that emerge from the interactions of neurons, the most interesting are the functions concerned with learning (the ability to modify behavior in response to experience) and with memory (the ability to store that modification over a period of time). Learning and memory are perhaps the most distinctive features of the mental processes of advanced animals, and these features reach their highest form in man. In fact, human beings are what they are in good measure because of what they have learned. It is therefore of theoretical importance, for the understanding of learning and for the study of behavioral evolution, to determine at what phylogenetic level of neuronal and behavioral organization one can begin to recognize aspects of the learning and memory processes that characterize human behavior. This determination is also of practical importance. The difficulty in studying the cellular mechanisms of memory in the brain of man or other mammals arises because such brains are immensely complex. For the human brain ethical issues also preclude this kind of study. It would therefore be congenial scientifically to be able to examine these processes effectively in simple systems.

It could be argued that the study of memory and learning as it relates to man cannot be pursued effectively in simple neuronal systems. The organization of the human brain seems so complex that trying to study human learning in a reduced form in simple neuronal systems is bound to fail. Man has intellectual abilities, a highly developed language and an ability for abstract thinking, which are not found in simpler animals and may require qualitatively different types of neuronal organization. Although such arguments have value, the critical question is not whether there is something special about the human brain. There clearly is. The question is rather what the human brain and human behavior have in common with the brain and the behavior of simpler animals. Where there are points of similarity they may involve common principles of brain organization that could profitably be studied in simple neural systems.

The answer to the question of similarity is clear. Ethologists such as Konrad Lorenz, Nikolaas Tinbergen and Karl von Frisch have shown that human beings share many common behavioral patterns with simpler animals, including elementary perception and motor coordination. The capacity to learn, in particular, is widespread; it has evolved in many invertebrate animals and in all vertebrates. The similarity of some of the learning processes suggests that the neuronal mechanisms for a given learning process may have features in common across phylogeny. For example, there appear to be no fundamental differences in structure, chemistry or function between the neurons and synapses in man and those of a squid, a snail or a leech. Consequently a complete and rigorous analysis of learning in such an invertebrate is likely to reveal mechanisms of general significance.

Simple invertebrates are attractive for such investigation because their nervous systems consist of between 10,000 and 100,000 cells, compared with the many billions in more complex animals. The cells are collected into discrete groups called ganglia, and each ganglion usually consists of between 500 and 1,500 neurons. This numerical simplification has made it possible to relate the function of individual cells directly to behavior. The result is a number of important findings that lead to a new way of looking at the relation between the brain and behavior.

The first major question that students of simple systems of neurons might examine is whether the various neurons of a region of the nervous system differ from one another. This question, which is central to an understanding of how behavior is mediated by the nervous system, was in dispute until recently. Some neurobiologists argued that the neurons of a brain are sufficiently similar in their properties to be regarded as identical units having interconnections of roughly equal value.

These arguments have now been strongly challenged, particularly by studies of invertebrates showing that many neurons can be individually identified and are invariant in every member of the species. The concept that neurons are unique was proposed as early as 1912 by the German biologist Richard Goldschmidt on the basis of his study of the nervous system of a primitive worm, the intestinal parasite *Ascaris.* The brain of this worm consists of several ganglia. When Goldschmidt examined the ganglia, he found they contained exactly 162 cells. The number never varied from animal to animal, and each cell always occupied a characteristic position. In spite of this clear-cut results Goldschmidt's work went largely unheeded.

More than 50 years later two groups at the Harvard Medical School returned to the problem independently. Masanori Otsuka, Edward A. Kravitz and David D. Potter, working with the lobster, and Wesley T. Frazier, Irving Kupfermann, Rafiq M. Waziri, Richard E. Coggeshall and I, working with the large marine snail *Aplysia,* found a similar but less complete invariance in the more complex nervous systems of these higher invertebrates. A comparable invariance was soon found in a variety of invertebrates, including the leech, the crayfish, the locust, the cricket and a number of snails. Here I shall limit myself to considering studies of *Aplysia,* particularly studies of a single ganglion: the abdominal ganglion. Similar findings have also emerged from the studies of other invertebrates.

In the abdominal ganglion of *Aplysia* neurons vary in size, position, shape, pigmentation, firing patterns and the chemical substances by which they transmit information to other cells. On the basis of such differences it is possible to recognize and name specific cells (R1, L1, R15 and so on). The firing patterns illustrate some of the differences. Certain cells are normally "silent" and others are spontaneously active. Among the active ones some fire regular action potentials, or nerve impulses, and others fire in recurrent brief bursts or trains. The different firing patterns have now been shown to result from differences in the types of ionic currents generated by the membrane of the cell body of the neurons. The cell-body membrane is quite different from the membrane of the axon, the long fiber of the neuron. When the membrane of the axon is active, it typi-

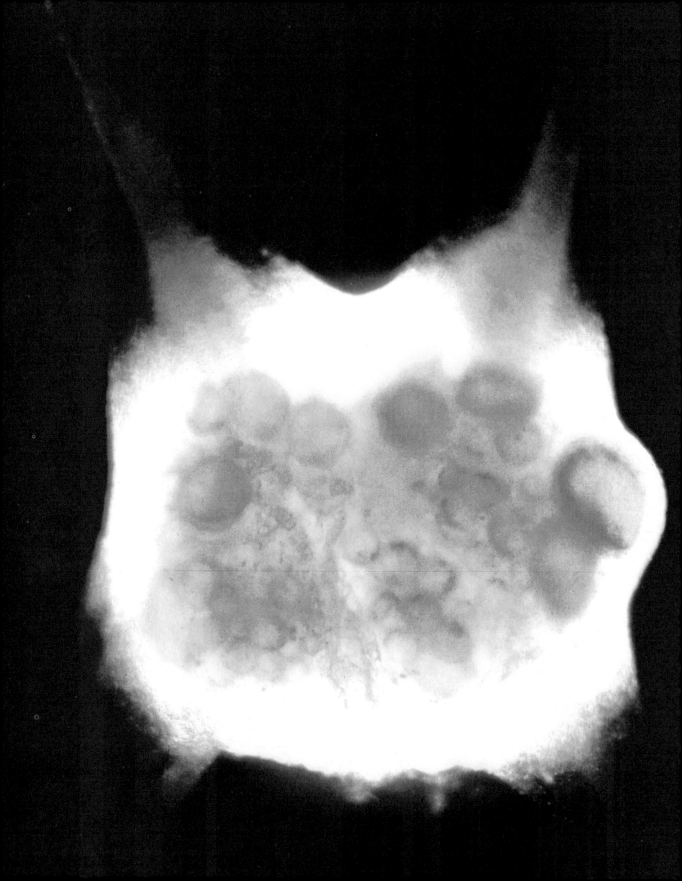

Figure 48 GROUP OF NEURONS from the dorsal surface of the abdominal ganglion of the snail *Aplysia*. The magnification is 90 diameters. A particularly large, dark brown neuron can be seen at the right side of the micrograph. It is the cell identified as R2 in Figure 49.

cally produces only an inflow of sodium ions and a delayed outflow of potassium ions, whereas the membrane of the cell body can produce six or seven distinct ionic currents that can flow in various combinations. Whether or not most cells in the mammalian nervous system are also unique individuals is not yet known.

The finding that neurons are invariant leads to further questions. Are the synaptic connections between cells also invariant? Does a given identified cell always connect to exactly the same follower cell

and not to others? A number of investigators have examined these questions in invertebrate animals and have found that cells indeed always make the same kinds of connections to other cells. The invariance applies not only to the connections but also to the "sign," or functional expression, of the connections, that is, whether they are excitatory or inhibitory.

Therefore Frazier, James E. Blankenship, Howard Wachtel and I next worked with identified cells to examine the rules that determine the functional expression of connections between cells. A single neuron has many branches and makes many connections. We asked: Are all the connections of a neuron specialized for inhibition or excitation, or can the firing of a neuron produce different actions at different branches? What determines whether a connection is excitatory or inhibitory? Is the sign of

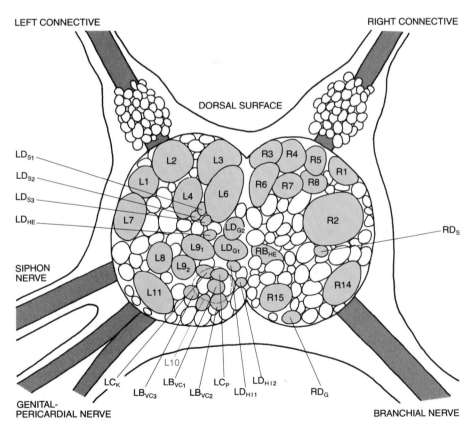

Figure 49 MAP OF ABDOMINAL GANGLION in *Aplysia californica*. Identified neurons are labeled L or R (for left or right hemiganglion) and assigned a number. Neurons that are members of a cluster, consisting of cells with simi- lar properties, are further identified by a cluster letter (LD) and a subscript representing the behavioral function of the neuron; such as HE for heart excitor and G1 and G2 for two gill motor neurons.

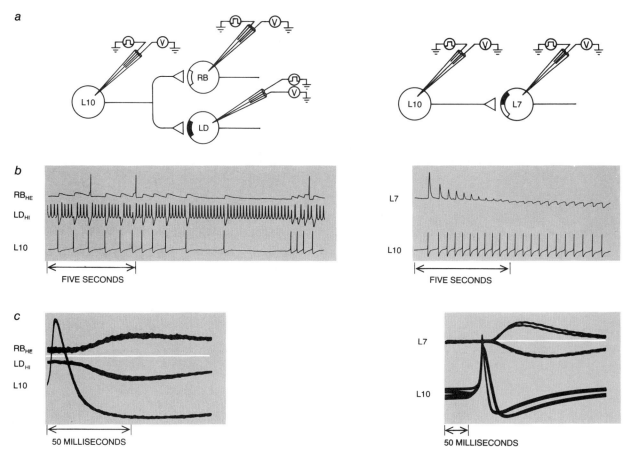

Figure 50 INVARIANCE OF CONNECTIONS between cells L10 and follower cells was ascertained (*a*) by stimulating and recording microelectrodes that were inserted in L10, a presynaptic neuron, and in three follower cells. L10 produces excitation (*white*) in RB, inhibition (*black*) in LD and both excitation and inhibition in L7. The respective firing patterns are shown in *b*. Superimposed sweeps (*at the left in c*) demonstrate constant latency between presynaptic spikes and the responses of two follower cells. Superposed traces from L10 and L7 (*at the right in c*) show that effect is excitatory (tall and narrow impulses) when L10 fires initially and inhibitory when it fires repeatedly (short and broad impulses).

the synaptic action determined by the chemical structure of the transmitter substance released by the presynaptic neuron, or is the nature of the postsynaptic receptor the determining factor? Does the neuron release the same transmitter from all its terminals?

One way to explore these questions is to look at the different connections made by a cell. The first cell we examined gave a clear answer: it mediated different actions through its various connections. The cell excited some follower cells, inhibited others and (perhaps most unexpectedly) made a dual con-

nection, which was both excitatory and inhibitory, to a third kind of cell. Moreover, it always excited precisely the same cells, always inhibited another specific group of cells and always made a dual connection with a third group. Its synaptic action could be accounted for by one transmitter substance: acetylcholine. The reaction of this substance with different types of receptors on the various follower cells determined whether the synaptic action would be excitatory or inhibitory.

The receptors determined the sign of the synaptic action by controlling different ionic channels in the membrane: primarily sodium for excitation and chloride for inhibition. The cells that received the dual connection had two types of receptor for the same transmitter, one receptor that controlled a sodium channel and another that controlled a chloride channel. The functional expression of chemical synaptic transmission is therefore determined by the types of receptor the follower cell has at a given postsynaptic site. (Similar results have been obtained by JacSue Kehoe of the École Normale in Paris, who has gone on to analyze in detail the properties of the various species of receptors to acetylcholine.) Thus, as was first suggested by Ladislav Tauc and Hersch Gerschenfeld of the Institute Marey in Paris, the chemical transmitter is only permissive; the instructive component of synaptic transmission is the nature of the receptor and the ionic channels it interacts with. This principle has proved to be fairly general. It applies to the neurons of vertebrates and invertebrates and to neurons utilizing various transmitters: acetylcholine, gamma-amino-butyric acid (GABA), serotonin, dopamine and histamine. (The principle also applies to the actions of certain peptide hormones on neurons, a subject to which I shall return.)

The discovery in invertebrate ganglia of identifiable cells that make precise connections with one another has led to the working out of the "wiring diagram" of various behavioral circuits and has therefore made possible an exact study of the causal relation of specific neurons to behavior. The term behavior refers to the observable actions of an organism. These range from complex acts such as talking or walking to simple acts such as the movement of a body part or a change in heart rate. Types of behavior that have been at least partly worked out in leeches, crayfishes and snails include feeding, various locomotor patterns and a variety of escape and defensive reactions.

The first finding to emerge from these studies is that individual cells exert a control over behavior that is specific and sometimes surprisingly powerful. The point can be illustrated by comparing the neural control of the heart in *Aplysia* with that in human beings.

The human heart beats spontaneously. Its intrinsic rhythm is neuronally modulated by the inhibitory action of cholinergic neurons (acetylcholine is the transmitter substance) with their axons in the vagus nerve and the excitatory action of noradrenergic neurons with their axons in the accelerator nerve. The modulation involves several thousand neurons. In *Aplysia* the heart also beats spontaneously; it is neuronally modulated by the inhibitory action of cholinergic neurons and the excitatory action of serotonergic neurons, but the modulation is accomplished by only four cells! Two cells excite the heart (only the "major excitor" cell is really important) and two inhibit it. Three other cells give rise to a constriction of the blood vessels and thereby control the animal's blood pressure.

Since individual cells connect invariably to the same follower cells and can mediate actions that have a different sign, certain cells at a critical point in the nervous system are in a position to control an entire behavioral sequence. As early as 1938 C. A. G. Wiersma, working with the crayfish at the California Institute of Technology, had appreciated the importance of single cells in behavior and had called them "command cells." Such cells have now been found in a variety of animals. A few of them have proved to be dual-action neurons. Hence John Koester, Earl M. Mayeri and I, working with *Aplysia* at the New York University School of Medicine, found that the dual-action neuron described above is a command cell for the neural circuit controlling the circulation. This one cell increases the rate and output of the heart by exciting the major cell that excites the heart while inhibiting the cells that inhibit the heart and the cells that constrict the major blood vessels. As a result of the increased activity of this one cell the heart beats faster and pumps more blood.

This is only a simple example of the behavioral functions of a command cell. In the crayfish and even in a more complex animal, the goldfish, a single impulse in a single command neuron causes the animal to flee from threatened danger. Recently Vernon Mountcastle of the Johns Hopkins University School of Medicine has suggested in this context that small groups of cells may serve similar command functions in the primate brain to control purposeful voluntary movements.

Hence a functional purpose of dual-action cells is to bring about a constellation of different physiological effects. A similar constellation can be achieved by the action of neuroendocrine cells, neurons that release hormones (the chemical substances that are usually carried in the bloodstream to act at distant sites). The abdominal ganglion of *Aplysia* contains two clusters of neuroendocrine cells, which are called bag cells because each cluster is bag-shaped. Kupfermann, working in our division at the Colum-

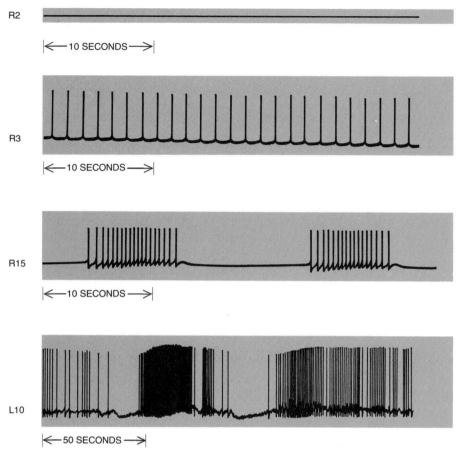

Figure 51 FIRING PATTERNS of identified neurons in *Aplysia*'s abdominal ganglion are portrayed. R2 is normally silent, R3 has a regular beating rhythm, R15 a regular bursting rhythm and L10 an irregular bursting rhythm. L10 is a command cell that controls other cells in the system.

bia University College of Physicians and Surgeons, has shown, as have Stephen Arch of Reed College and Felix Strumwasser and his colleagues at Cal Tech, that the bag cells release a polypeptide hormone that controls egg laying. Mayeri has found that this hormone has long-lasting actions on various cells in the abdominal ganglion, exciting some and inhibiting others.

One of the cells excited by this hormone is the dual-action command cell that controls the heart rate. As a result the heart speeds up to provide the extra flow of blood to the tissues that the animal requires during egg laying. Thus superimposed on a precise pattern of connections that provide short-range interaction of neurons is an equally precise pattern of long-range interactions achieved by the hormones released by neuroendocrine cells. The

precise effect of each hormone seems to be determined, as synaptic effects are, by the nature of the receptors on the target cells.

The finding that behavior is mediated by invariant cells interconnecting in precise and invariant ways might suggest that simple animals differ from more complex ones in having stereotyped and fixed repertoires of activity. It is not so. Studies in different invertebrates have shown that behavior in simple animals is quite capable of being modified by learning.

We have explored this subject most fully in one of *Aplysia*'s simplest kinds of behavior: a defensive reflex action in which the gill is withdrawn after a stimulus. The gill is in a respiratory chamber called the mantle cavity. The chamber is covered by a protective sheet, the mantle shelf, that terminates in

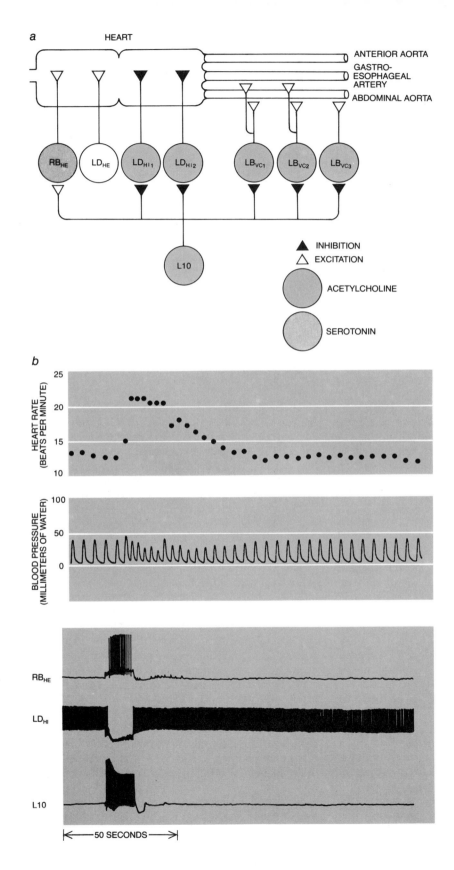

Figure 52 BEHAVIORAL CONTROL by the single neuron L10 is shown by its effect on cardiovascular motor neurons of *Aplysia*. L10 makes synaptic connections (*a*) with six of the cells; the color of each cell indicates what chemical transmitter it utilizes. The activity of L10 (*b*) increases heart rate and blood pressure by exciting RB_{HE} and inhibiting LD_{HI}.

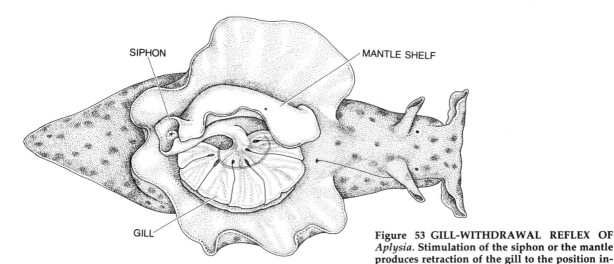

SIPHON

MANTLE SHELF

GILL

Figure 53 GILL-WITHDRAWAL REFLEX OF *Aplysia.* **Stimulation of the siphon or the mantle produces retraction of the gill to the position indicated in color.**

a fleshy spout, the siphon. When a weak or a moderately intense stimulus is applied to the siphon, the gill contracts and withdraws into the mantle cavity. This reflex is analogous to the withdrawal responses found in almost all higher animals, such as the one in which a human being jerks a hand away from a hot object. *Aplysia* and the other animals exhibit two forms of learning with such reflexes: habituation and sensitization.

Habituation is a decrease in the strength of a behavioral response that occurs when an initially novel stimulus is presented repeatedly. When an animal is presented with a novel stimulus, it at first responds with a combination of orienting and defensive reflexes. With repeated stimulation the animal readily learns to recognize the stimulus. If the stimulus proves to be unrewarding or innocuous, the animal will reduce and ultimately suppress its responses to it. Although habituation is remarkably simple, it is probably the most widespread of all forms of learning. Through habituation animals, including human beings, learn to ignore stimuli that have lost novelty or meaning; habituation frees them to attend to stimuli that are rewarding or significant for survival. Habituation is thought to be the first learning process to emerge in human infants and is commonly utilized to study the development of intellectual processes such as attention, perception and memory.

An interesting aspect of habituation in vertebrates is that it gives rise to both short- and long-term

memory and has therefore been employed to explore the relation between the two. Thomas J. Carew, Harold M. Pinsker and I found that a similar relation holds for *Aplysia*. After a single training session of from 10 to 15 tactile stimuli to the siphon the withdrawal reflex habituates. The memory for the stimulus is short-lived; partial recovery can be detected within an hour and almost complete recovery generally occurs within a day. Recovery in this type of learning is equivalent to forgetting. As with the repetition of more complex learning tasks, however, four repeated training sessions of only 10 stimuli each produce profound habituation and a memory for the stimulus that lasts for weeks.

The first question that Vincent Castellucci, Kupfermann, Pinsker and I asked was: What are the loci and mechanisms of short-term habituation? The neural circuit controlling gill withdrawal is quite simple. A stimulus to the skin of the siphon activates the 24 sensory neurons there; they make direct connections to six motor cells in the gill, and the motor cells connect directly to the muscle. The sensory neurons also excite several interneurons, which are interposed neurons.

By examining these cells during habituation we found that short-term habituation involved a change in the strength of the connection made by the sensory neurons on their central target cells: the interneurons and the motor neurons. This localization was most fortunate, because now we could examine what happened during habituation simply by analyzing the changes in two cells, the presynaptic sensory neuron and the postsynaptic motor neuron, and in the single set of connections between them.

The strength of a connection can be studied by recording the synaptic action produced in the motor cells by an individual sensory neuron. It is possible to simulate the habituation training session of from 10 to 15 stimuli by stimulating a sensory neuron following the exact time sequence used for the in-

tact animal. The stimulus can be adjusted so that it generates a single action potential. The first time the neuron is caused to fire an action potential it produces a highly effective synaptic action, which is manifested as a large excitatory postsynaptic potential in the motor cell. The subsequent action potentials initiated in the sensory neuron during a training session give rise to progressively smaller excitatory postsynaptic potentials. This depression

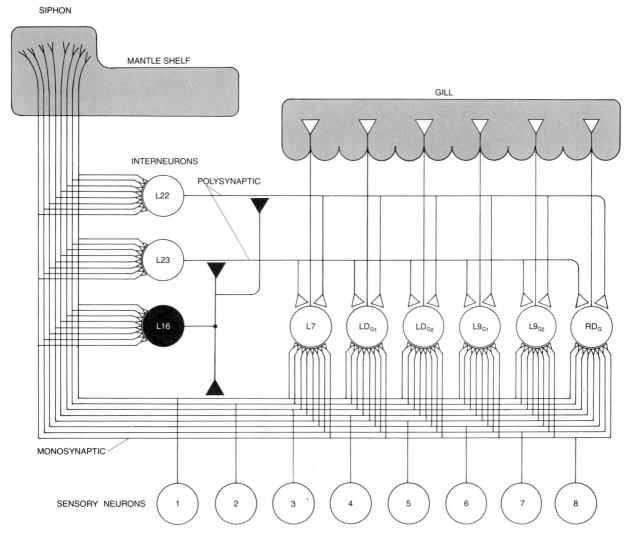

Figure 54 NEURAL CIRCUITRY of a behavioral reflex of *Aplysia,* the gill-withdrawal reflex, is depicted schematically. The animal withdraws its gill when the siphon on the mantle is stimulated. The skin of the siphon is innervated by about 24 sensory neurons (only eight are shown). The sensory neurons connect to six identified gill motor neurons, L7 to RD_G, and to one inhibitory cell (L16) and two interposed excitatory interneurons (L22 and L23) which contact motor neurons.

in the effectiveness of the connection parallels and accounts for the behavioral habituation. As with the behavior, the synaptic depression resulting from a single training session persists for more than an hour. Following a second training session there is a more pronounced depression of the synaptic potential, and further training sessions can depress the synaptic potential completely.

What causes the changes in the strength of the synaptic connection? Do they involve a change in the presynaptic sensory neuron, reflecting a decrease in the release of the transmitter substance, or a change in the postsynaptic cell, reflecting a decrease in the sensitivity of the receptors to the chemical transmitter? The questions can be answered by analyzing changes in the amplitude of the synaptic potential in terms of its quantal components.

As was first shown by José del Castillo and Bernhard Katz at University College London, transmitter is released not as single molecules but as "quanta," or multimolecular packets. Each packet contains roughly the same amount of transmitter (several thousand molecules). The quanta are thought to be stored in subcellular organelles called synaptic vesicles that are seen in abundance at synaptic endings examined with the electronic microscope. Since the number of transmitter molecules in each quantum does not ordinarily change, the number of quanta released by each action potential is a fairly reliable index of the total amount of transmitter released. Each quantum in turn produces a miniature excitatory postsynaptic potential of characteristic size in the postsynaptic cell. The size is an indication of how sensitive the postsynaptic receptors are to the several thousand molecules of transmitter released by each packet.

Castellucci and I, working with *Aplysia*, found that the decrease in the amplitude of the synaptic action potential with habituation was paralleled by a decrease in the number of chemical quanta released. In contrast, the size of the miniature postsynaptic potential did not change, indicating that there was no change in the sensitivity of the postsynaptic receptor. The results show that the site of short-term habituation is the presynaptic terminals of the sensory neurons and that the mechanism of habituation is a progressive decrease in the amount of transmitter released by the sensory-neuron terminals onto their central target cells. Studies in the crayfish by Robert S. Zucker of the University of

California at Berkeley and by Franklin B. Krasne of the University of California at Los Angeles and in the cat by Paul B. Farel and Richard F. Thompson of the University of California at Irvine indicate that this mechanism may be quite general.

What is responsible for the decrease in the number of quanta released by each action potential? The number is largely determined by the concentration of free calcium in the presynaptic terminal. Calcium is one of three kinds of ion involved in the generation of each action potential in the terminal. The depolarizing upstroke of the action potential is produced mainly by the inflow of sodium ions into the terminal, but it also involves a lesser and delayed flow of calcium ions. The repolarizing downstroke is largely produced by the outflow of potassium ions. The inflow of calcium is essential for the release of transmitter. Calcium is thought to enable the synaptic vesicles to bind to release sites in the presynaptic terminals. This binding is a critical step preliminary to the release of transmitter from the vesicles (the process termed exocytosis). It therefore seems possible that the amount of calcium coming into the terminals with each action potential is not fixed but is variable and that the amount might be modulated by habituation.

The best way to examine changes in the flow of calcium into terminals would be to record from the terminals directly. We have been unable to do so because the terminals are very small. Because the properties of the calcium channels of the cell body resemble those of the terminals, however, one of our graduate students, Marc Klein, set about examining the change in the calcium current of the cell body that accompanies the synaptic depression.

The calcium current turns on slowly during the action potential and so is normally overlapped by the potassium current. To unmask the calcium current we exposed the ganglion to tetraethylammonium (TEA), an agent that selectively blocks some of the delayed potassium current. By blocking the repolarizing action of the potassium current the agent produces a significant increase in the duration of the action potential. Much of this prolongation is due to the unopposed action of the calcium current. The duration of the action potential prolonged by TEA is a good assay for changes in calcium current.

We next examined the release of transmitter by the terminals of the sensory neurons, as measured by the size of the synaptic potential in the motor cell, and the changes recorded simultaneously in the calcium current, as measured by the duration of the action potential. We found that repeated stimulation of the sensory neuron at rates that produce habituation led to a progressive decrease in the duration of the calcium component of the action potential that paralleled the decrease in the release of transmitter. Spontaneous recovery of the synaptic potential and of the behavior were accompanied by an increase in the calcium current.

W hat we have learned so far about the mechanisms of short-term habituation indicates that this type of learning involves a modulation in the strength of a previously existing synaptic connection. The strength of the connection is determined by the amount of transmitter released, which is in turn controlled by the degree to which an action potential in the presynaptic terminal can acti-

vate the calcium current. The storage of the memory for short-term habituation therefore resides in the persistence, over minutes and hours, of the depression in the calcium current in the presynaptic terminal.

What are the limits of this change? How much can the effectiveness of a given synapse change as a result of learning, and how long can such changes endure? I have mentioned that repeated training sessions can completely depress the synaptic connections between the sensory and the motor cells. Can this condition be maintained? Can long-term habituation give rise to a complete and prolonged inactivation of a previously functioning synapse?

These questions bear on the long-standing debate among students of learning about the relation of short- and long-term memory. The commonly ac-

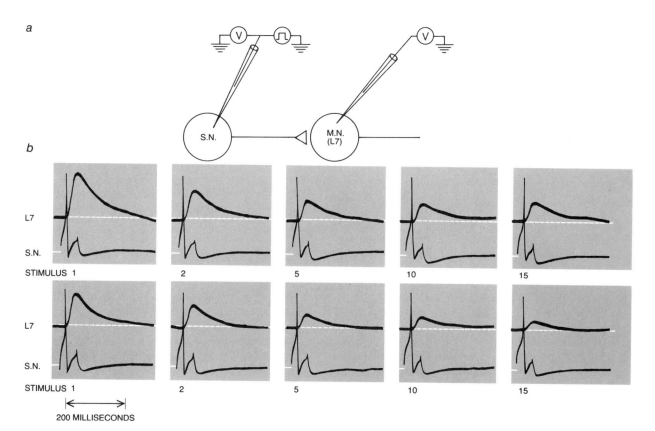

Figure 55 HABITUATION PROCESS. An animal's response to a stimulus gradually declines if the stimulus is unimportant. This is an elementary form of learning and memory that can be seen at the level of the single neuron. A sensory neuron (S.N.) from *Aplysia* that synapses on motor neuron L7 is set up to be stimulated every 10 seconds (*a*). Records from two consecutive training sessions of 15 stimuli (*b*) show that the response of L7 declines and vanishes.

cepted idea is that the two kinds of memory involve different memory processes. This idea is based, however, on rather indirect evidence.

Castellucci, Carew and I set out to examine the hypothesis more directly by comparing the effectiveness of the connections made by the population of sensory neurons on an identified gill motor cell, L7, in four groups of *Aplysia:* untrained animals that served as controls, and groups examined respectively one day, one week and three weeks after long-term habituation training. We found that in the control animals about 90 percent of the sensory neurons made extremely effective connections to L7, whereas in the animals examined one day and one week after long-term habituation the figure was 30 percent. Even in the three-week group only about 60 percent of the cells made detectable connections to L7. Here, then, are previously effective synaptic connections that become inactive and remain that way for more than a week as a result of a simple learning experience.

Hence whereas short-term habituation involves a transient decrease in synaptic efficacy, long-term habituation produces a more prolonged and profound change, leading to a functional disruption of most of the previously effective connections. The data are interesting for three reasons: (1) they provide direct evidence that a specific instance of long-term memory can be explained by a long-term change in synaptic effectiveness, (2) they show that surprisingly little training is needed to produce a profound change in synaptic transmission at synapses critically involved in learning, and (3) they make clear that short- and long-term habituation can share a common neuronal locus, namely the synapses the sensory neurons make on the motor neurons. Short- and long-term habituation also involve aspects of the same cellular mechanism: a depression of excitatory transmission. One now needs to determine whether the long-term synaptic depression is presynaptic and whether it involves an inactivation of the calcium current. If it does, it would support on a more fundamental level the notion that short- and long-term memory can involve a single memory trace.

Sensitization is a slightly more complex form of learning that can be seen in the gill-withdrawal reflex. It is the prolonged enhancement of an animal's preexisting response to a stimulus as a result of the presentation of a second stimulus that is noxious. Whereas habituation requires an animal to learn to ignore a particular stimulus because its consequences are trivial, sensitization requires the animal to learn to attend to a stimulus because it is accompanied by potentially painful or dangerous consequences. Therefore when an *Aplysia* is presented with a noxious stimulus to the head, the gill-withdrawal reflex response to a repeated stimulus to the siphon is greatly enhanced. As with habituation, sensitization can last from minutes to days and weeks, depending on the amount of training. Here I shall focus only on the short-term form.

Castellucci and I found that sensitization entails an alteration of synaptic transmission at the same locus that is involved in habituation: the synapses made by the sensory neurons on their central target cells. Our physiological studies and subsequent morphological studies by Craig Bailey, Mary C. Chen and Robert Hawkins indicate that the neurons mediating sensitization end near the synaptic terminals of the sensory neurons and enhance the release of transmitter by increasing the number of quanta turned loose by each action potential in the sensory neuron. The process is therefore called presynaptic facilitation. It is interesting because it illustrates (as does the earlier finding of presynaptic inhibition in another system by Joseph Dudel and Stephen Kuffler of the Harvard Medical School) that neurons have receptors to transmitters at two quite different sites. Receptors on the cell body and on the dendrites determine whether a cell should fire an action potential, and receptors on the synaptic terminals determine how much transmitter each action potential will release.

The same locus—the presynaptic terminals of the sensory neurons—can therefore be regulated in opposite ways by opposing forms of learning. It can be depressed as a result of the intrinsic activity within the neuron that occurs with habituation, and it can be facilitated by sensitization as a result of the activity of other neurons that synapse on the terminals. These findings at the level of the single cell support the observation at the behavioral level that habituation and sensitization are independent and opposing forms of learning.

This finding raises an interesting question. Sensitization can enhance a normal reflex response, but can it counteract the profound depression in the reflex produced by long-term habituation? If it can, does it restore the completely inactivated synaptic connections produced by long-term habituation? Carew, Castellucci and I examined this question and found that sensitization reversed the depressed be-

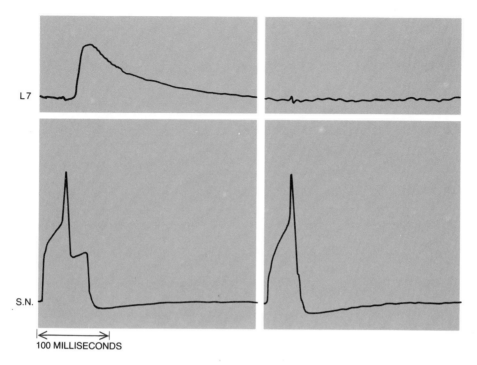

L7

S.N.

|← 100 MILLISECONDS →|

Figure 56 LONG TERM HABITUATION is shown in a comparison of synaptic connections between a sensory neuron (S.N.) and the motor neuron L7 in untrained *Aply-*sia (*left*), which served as controls, and in *Aplysia* **that received long-term habituation training (*right*).**

havior. Moreover, the synapses that were functionally inactivated (and would have remained so for weeks) were restored within an hour by a sensitizing stimulus to the head.

Hence there are synaptic pathways in the brain that are determined by developmental processes but that, being predisposed to learning, can be functionally inactivated and reactivated by experience. In fact, at these modifiable synapses a rather modest amount of training or experience is necessary to produce profound changes. If the finding were applicable to the human brain, it would imply that even during simple social experiences, as when two people speak with each other, the action of the neuronal machinery in one person's brain is capable of having a direct and perhaps long-lasting effect on the modifiable synaptic connections in the brain of the other.

Short-term sensitization is particularly attractive from an experimental point of view because it promises to be amenable to biochemical analysis. As a first step Hawkins, Castellucci and I have identified specific cells in the abdominal ganglion of

Aplysia that produce presynaptic facilitation. By injecting an electron-dense marker substance to fill the cell and label its synaptic endings we found that the endings contain vesicles resembling those found in *Aplysia* by Ludmiela Shkolnik and James H. Schwartz in a neuron whose transmitter had previously been established to be serotonin. Consistent with the possible serotonergic nature of this cell, Marcello Brunelli, Castellucci, Tom Tomosky-Sykes and I found that serotonin enhanced the monosynaptic connection between the sensory neuron and the motor cell L7, whereas other likely transmitters did not.

We next uncovered an interesting link between serotonin and the intracellular messenger cyclic adenosine monophosphate (cyclic AMP). It has been known since the classic work of Earl W. Sutherland, Jr., and his colleagues at Vanderbilt University that most peptide hormones do not enter the target cell but instead act on a receptor on the cell surface to stimulate an enzyme called adenylate cyclase that catalyzes the conversion in the cell of adenosine triphosphate (ATP) into cyclic AMP,

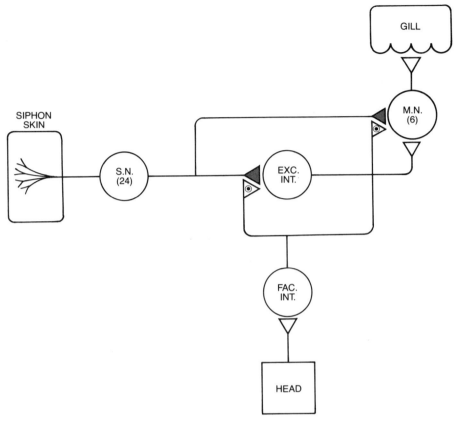

Figure 57 SENSITIZATION. The gill-withdrawal reflex of *Aplysia* **is intensified because of a noxious stimulus to the head. This stimulus activates facilitating interneurons, which end on the synaptic terminals of the sensory** neurons. **Those interneurons are capable of changing the effectiveness of their synapses. The transmitter of the facilitating interneurons is thought to be serotonin (***circled dots***).**

which then acts as a "second messenger" (the hormone is the first messenger) at several points inside the cell to initiate a set of appropriate changes in function.

Howard Cedar, Schwartz and I found that strong and prolonged stimulation of the pathway from the head that mediates sensitization in *Aplysia* gave rise to a synaptically mediated increase in cyclic AMP in the entire ganglion. Cedar and Schwartz and Irwin Levitan and Samuel Barondes also found that they could generate a prolonged increase in cyclic AMP by incubating the ganglion with serotonin. To explore the relation between serotonin and cyclic AMP, Brunelli, Castellucci and I injected cyclic AMP intracellularly into the cell body of the sensory neuron and found that it also produced presynaptic facilitation, whereas injection of 5'-AMP (the

breakdown product of cyclic AMP) or still another second messenger, cyclic GMP, did not.

Since habituation involves a decrease in calcium current, it was attractive to think that cyclic AMP might exert its facilitating actions by increasing the calcium current. As I have mentioned, the calcium current is normally masked by the potassium current. Klein and I therefore examined action potentials in the sensory neurons with the potassium current reduced by TEA. Stimulating the pathway from the head that mediates sensitization or a single facilitating neuron enhanced the calcium current, as was evident in the increased duration of the action potential in TEA, and the enhancement persisted for 15 minutes or longer. The increase in calcium current paralleled the enhanced transmitter release, and both synaptic changes in turn paralleled the increase in the reflex response to a sensitizing stimulus.

The enhancement of the calcium current, as it is seen in the prolongation of the calcium component of the action potential after stimulation of the sensitizing pathway, could be produced by extracellular application of either serotonin or two substances that increase the intracellular level of cyclic AMP by inhibiting phosphodiesterase, the enzyme that breaks down cyclic AMP. Similar effects were observed after direct intracellular injection of cyclic AMP, but not of 5'-AMP.

On the basis of these results Klein and I have proposed that stimulation of the facilitating neurons of the sensitizing pathway leads to the release of serotonin, which activates a serotonin-sensitive enzyme (adenylate cyclase) in the membrane of the sensory-neuron terminal. The resulting increase in cyclic AMP in the terminal leads to a greater activation of the calcium current either directly by activation of the calcium channel or indirectly by a decrease in an opposing potassium current. With each action potential the influx of calcium rises and more transmitter is released.

The availability of large cells whose electrical properties and interconnections can be thoroughly studied was the major initial attraction for using *Aplysia* to study behavior. The size of these cells might now prove to be an even greater advantage for exploring the subcellular and biochemical mechanisms of learning on the one hand and possible changes in membrane structure on the other. For example, it will be interesting to see more precisely how the increase in the level of cyclic AMP during sensitization is linked to the activation of a calcium current, because the linkage could provide the first step toward a molecular understanding of this simple form of short-term learning.

A number of mechanisms come to mind. The channels through which ions traverse the neuronal membranes are thought to consist of protein molecules. An obvious possibility is therefore that cyclic AMP activates one or more protein kinases, enzymes that Paul Greengard of the Yale University School of Medicine has suggested may provide a common molecular mechanism for mediating the various actions of cyclic AMP within the cell. Protein kinases are enzymes that phosphorylate proteins, that is, they link a phosphoryl group to a side chain of the amino acids serine or threonine in the protein molecule, thereby changing the charge and configuration of proteins and altering their function, activating some and inactivating others. Phosphorylation could serve as an effective mechanism for the regulation of memory. One way sensitization

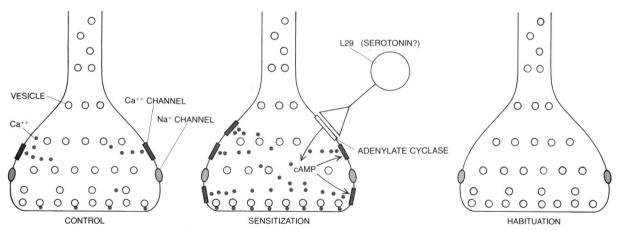

Figure 58 SHORT-TERM SENSITIZATION AND HABITUATION. In a control situation (*left*) a cell fires before either sensitization or habituation has set in. Calcium channels (Ca^{++}) and sodium channels (Na^+) are opened. Sensitization is triggered by cell group L29 probably releasing serotonin. Adenylate cyclase catalyzes cyclic AMP in the neuron terminals, which increases the influx of calcium ions, thereby increasing transmitter release. In habituation repeated impulses probably decrease the number of operating calcium channels, leading to a decrease in transmitter release.

might work is that the calcium-channel protein becomes activated (or the opposing potassium-channel protein becomes inactivated) when it is phosphorylated by a protein kinase that is dependent on cyclic AMP.

Sensitization holds an interesting position in the hierarchy of learning. It is frequently considered to be a precursor form of classical conditioning. In both sensitization and classical conditioning a reflex response to a stimulus is enhanced as a result of the activation of another pathway. Sensitization differs from conditioning in being nonassociative; the sensitizing stimulus is effective in enhancing reflex responsiveness whether or not it is paired in time with the reflex stimulus. Several types of associative learning have now been demonstrated in mollusks by Alan Gelperin of Princeton University, by George Mpitsos and Stephen Collins of Case Western Reserve University and by Terry Crow and Daniel L. Alkon of the National Institutes of Health. Recently Terry Walters, Carew and I have obtained evidence for associative conditioning in *Aplysia*. We may therefore soon be in a position to analyze precisely how the mechanisms of sensitization relate to those of associative learning.

Another direction that research can now take is to examine the relation between the initial development of the neural circuit in the embryo and its later modification by learning. Both development and learning involve functional changes in the nervous system: changes in the effectiveness of synapses and in other properties of neurons. How are such changes related? Are the mechanisms of learning based on those of developmental plasticity, or do completely new processes specialized for learning emerge later?

Whatever the answers to these intriguing questions may be, the surprising and heartening thing that has emerged from the study of invertebrate animals is that one can now pinpoint and observe at the cellular level, and perhaps ultimately at the molecular level, simple aspects of memory and learning. Although certain higher mental activities are characteristic of the complex brains of higher animals, it is now clear that elementary aspects of what are regarded as mental processes can be found in the activity of just a very few neurons. It will therefore be interesting both philosophically and technically to see to what degree complex forms of mentation can be explained in terms of simpler components and mechanisms. To the extent that such reductionist explanations are possible it will also be important to determine how the units of this elementary alphabet of mentation are combined to yield the language of much more complex mental processes.

POSTSCRIPT

The study of the cellular basis for learning has moved in the past decade to the search for the molecular basis for neuronal plasticity. Indeed, work on neurophysiology of memory and learning has focused, in recent years, on the unveiling of the molecular mechanism that underlies the modulation of synaptic and electroresponsive aspects of neuronal functions. The study of the effect of second messengers, of protein phosphorylation and, ultimately, of the regulation of gene expression on single-cell electrophysiology is the main impetus in the progression toward understanding short- and long-term memory. While this field is still very new, research in simple invertebrate preparations has been seminal in forcing other neuroscientists to consider the mechanism by which information is stored and retrieved in other living forms. The reader is referred to two reviews on this subject (see Goelet et al., 1986 and Neary, 1986).

The Chemical Differentiation of Nerve Cells

The development of the intricate network of nerve cells that makes up the nervous system requires each cell to "choose" a transmitter substance appropriate to its specific connections with other cells.

• • •

Paul H. Patterson, David D. Potter and Edwin J. Furshpan

July, 1978

The flow of information through the nervous system is determined by the particular pattern of connections made by the neurons, or nerve cells, with one another and with other body tissues such as muscles and glands. How this vastly complex network is established during the development of the organism is a basic and intriguing question. In the embryo the initially separated neurons make contact partly by migrating and partly by sending out the thin extensions of the cell body called axons and dendrites. These fibers usually branch repeatedly and may project to distant parts of the nervous system or leave the nervous system to innervate effector tissues. The site of communication between two neurons or between a neuron and an effector cell is the synapse. Here the axon terminal of the innervating neuron comes very close to the target cell but does not quite touch it; the intervening gap is filled with fluid and is called the synaptic cleft. On the arrival of a nerve impulse molecules of a neurotransmitter chemical are released from the terminal, travel across the synaptic cleft and combine with highly specific receptor proteins on the surface of the target cell. The activation of the receptors by the neurotransmitter triggers an electrical or biochemical response.

The fact that both chemistry and topology are involved in the architecture of the nervous system provides the system with an order of complexity beyond that of the man-made circuitry of computers. More than a dozen different substances are thought to be neurotransmitters, and they can be either excitatory (making the target cell more active) or inhibitory (preventing the target cell from becoming active). How do neurons in the developing nervous system "decide" which neurotransmitter to secrete in accordance with their location and function? And how is the synapse formed so that there is an appropriate match between the neurotransmitter secreted by the innervating neuron and the receptors present on the target cell? The investigation of these questions has involved the collaboration of electrophysiologists, biochemists and electron microscopists in several laboratories.

In our laboratory at the Harvard Medical School we and 14 colleagues have approached the general problem of how neurons differentiate chemically by examining the development of the autonomic nervous system, which regulates the activities of the circulatory system and a variety of organs and glands. The advantage of this system for such work is that its peripheral portions are readily accessible to the investigator. Moreover, the autonomic nervous system's chemical organization is relatively simple: most of its constituent nerve cells secrete either acetylcholine or norepinephrine (noradrenalin); they are respectively termed cholinergic or adrenergic. It seems reasonable to assume that the basic mechanisms involved in the decision of an autonomic neuron to become either cholinergic or adrenergic are analogous to those that determine which of several possible neurotransmitters will be secreted by a neuron in the brain.

There are two major types of pathway in the autonomic nervous system: sympathetic and parasympathetic (see Figure 59). These two subsystems often have antagonistic actions on the same organ. For example, the muscle cells of the heart, which contract spontaneously and rhythmically, are innervated by both sympathetic and parasympathetic nerves. In situations of stress the sympathetic

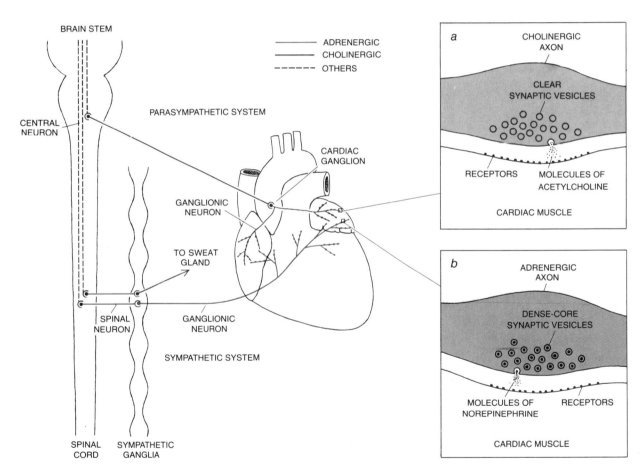

Figure 59 TWO AUTONOMIC PATHWAYS control the frequency of the heart beat. When the sympathetic system is active, reflex pathways excite sympathetic neurons in the spinal cord; these project to ganglionic neurons, which are excited and make the heart beat faster by secreting norepinephrine onto the cardiac muscle cells. When the parasympathetic system is active, reflex pathways excite parasympathetic neurons in the medulla, which project to target neurons in the cardiac ganglion that make the heart beat more slowly by secreting acetylcholine. Secretion of neurotransmitter takes place at varicosities, small swellings at intervals along the adrenergic and cholinergic axons (*insets right*).

nerves secrete norepinephrine, which makes the heart beat faster and more strongly. In periods of calm or inactivity the parasympathetic nerves secrete acetylcholine, which makes the heart beat slower.

Both autonomic pathways innervating the heart begin with neurons in the brain or spinal cord. These central neurons do not project directly to the heart muscle but make excitatory cholinergic synapses on neurons in a ganglion, a way station outside the spinal cord; the ganglionic neurons in turn innervate the heart muscle. The sympathetic pathway therefore consists of a cholinergic central neuron and an adrenergic ganglionic neuron, both of which are excitatory; the parasympathetic pathway consists of a cholinergic central neuron and a cholinergic ganglionic neuron, the former excitatory and the latter inhibitory. (The ability of acetylcholine to excite at the first synapse and inhibit at the second synapse is due to differences in the chemistry of the target cells.) Clearly the normal control of the heart depends on the ability of the neurons in the two autonomic pathways to secrete the correct neurotransmitter. For example, if the ganglionic sympathetic neurons secreted acetylcholine instead of norepinephrine, the heart would be inappropriately inhibited.

What determines whether a given neuron in an autonomic pathway will become cholinergic or adrenergic? In investigating this question we and our colleagues have done most of our experiments on immature neurons obtained from sympathetic ganglia of newborn rats and grown in tissue culture. This preparation was chosen for three reasons. First, the adult sympathetic ganglion contains both adrenergic neurons and a smaller number of cholinergic neurons (which innervate certain blood vessels and sweat glands), so that the differentiation of the two types of neuron can be studied in the same system. Second, as has been demonstrated by Rita Levi-Montalcini and her colleagues at Washington University, the normal development of sympathetic neurons in the intact animal depends on the presence of a particular protein named nerve-growth factor (NGF). When NGF is added to the culture medium, sympathetic neurons can be grown in culture.

Dennis Bray, who is now at the Medical Research Council Cell Biophysics Unit in London, later discovered specific culture conditions in which sympathetic neurons of the newborn rat survive but the non-neuronal cells of the ganglion die off. In this instance the sympathetic neurons develop in the virtual absence of any other cell type. Third, when neurons are removed from the sympathetic ganglia of the newborn rat, they are still immature in many basic respects: most of them have not made synaptic connections and are at an early stage in the differentiation of neurotransmitter metabolism.

The advantage of studying the development of neurons in culture rather than in the intact animal is that the investigator has better control over the cellular and fluid environment of the neurons and can thereby more readily investigate the factors crucial for the induction or control of particular cellular functions. Of course, the cultured neurons must be supplied with nutrients that they would normally receive from the blood, such as amino acids, sugars and vitamins. The proper balance of oxygen and carbon dioxide, normally maintained by the lungs, is accomplished by gas exchange between the culture medium and the controlled environment of the culture incubator. The removal of toxic wastes, normally achieved by the kidney, is assumed by the periodic replacement of the culture medium. Because the isolated cells have no immunological defenses against microorganisms, the instruments, dishes and mediums must be sterile. Finally, in order to enhance the adherence of the axons and dendrites to the substrate, the plastic surface of the culture dish is coated with a thin film of collagen, a natural constituent of the intercellular matrix.

In the presence of NGF, but not in its absence, the sympathetic neurons survive and grow extensions that continue to elongate for many weeks. Eventually the surface of the dish becomes covered with a dense meshwork of axons and dendrites. Surprisingly the neurons that are grown in this highly artificial environment in the absence of non-neuronal cells acquire many of the characteristics of normal sympathetic neurons and do so on a time course similar to the one observed in the intact animal. The cultured neurons generate impulses, possess surface receptors for acetylcholine (the transmitter released by the central neurons that normally innervate them) and develop the ability to manufacture norepinephrine from its amino acid precursor, tyrosine. Indeed, most if not all of the neurons in sympathetic ganglia manufacture norepinephrine before the rat is born. These findings suggest that before the neurons were removed from the animal they received developmental signals that instructed them to utilize norepinephrine as a transmitter. In

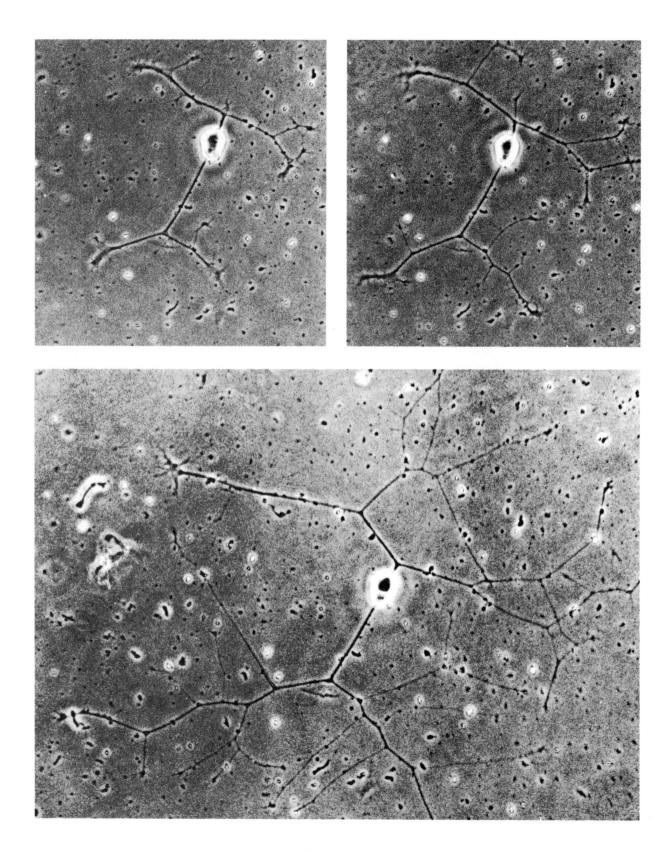

the presence of NGF, which allows the cells to survive in culture, they simply read out the appropriate genetic program.

In the absence of non-neuronal cells the cultured sympathetic neurons also form synapses with one another. As has been shown by Richard P. Bunge and his colleagues at the Washington University School of Medicine, these synapses structurally resemble those made by adult adrenergic neurons in that the norepinephrine is stored in tiny vesicles, or sacs, that have dense cores when they are stained with permanganate for electron microscopy. Although norepinephrine is released and taken up at these synapses, the neurotransmitter does not have any detectable effect on the electrical activity of the target neuron, meaning that either the cultured neurons do not possess receptors for norepinephrine or, if receptors are present, they fail to evoke a significant electrical signal. The existence of such electrically silent synapses is quite unusual, and few other instances are known.

When the sympathetic neurons are cultured together with non-neuronal cells from the ganglion, striking differences in the chemical differentiation of the neurons are observed. Instead of expressing only adrenergic functions, as they do in the absence of the non-neuronal cells, the mixed cultures manufacture and accumulate high levels of acetylcholine, indicating that many of the neurons have become cholinergic. Electrophysiological investigation has revealed that a substantial fraction of the neurons also form cholinergic synapses with their neighbors, thereby substituting for the normal cholinergic input from the central neurons, which are absent from the culture. Unlike the electrically silent adrenergic synapses formed in the absence of non-neuronal cells, these cholinergic synapses are electrically active and excitatory.

Is the effect of the non-neuronal cells on the choice of transmitter exerted by way of direct contact with the sympathetic neurons, or rather by the release of some chemical factor into the culture medium? To answer this question we grew the neurons in one set of dishes and the non-neuronal cells in another set. Every two days the medium that had been "conditioned" by incubating it with the non-neuronal cells was transferred to the neuronal cultures. We found that treatment with conditioned medium was sufficient to induce cholinergic properties in the sympathetic neurons: the cells synthesized and accumulated acetylcholine and secreted it at functional cholinergic synapses with one another.

The effect of conditioned medium was dose-dependent: the greater the amount that was added to the growth medium of the neurons, the more acetylcholine the cells made and the more likely they were to form cholinergic synapses with one another. At the same time the neurons made less norepinephrine and fewer adrenergic synapses. Thus in the population of neurons as a whole the expression of cholinergic functions was roughly reciprocal to the expression of adrenergic functions. Moreover, the differentiation of cholinergic metabolism in the presence of conditioned medium had a time course similar to that of adrenergic metabolism in the absence of conditioned medium. We have recently obtained evidence that the active ingredient of conditioned medium is a large molecule, and attempts to purify it are now under way.

How does this developmental factor released by non-neuronal cells influence the choice of neurotransmitter? One possibility is that at the outset there are two populations of neurons, one predestined to become adrenergic and the other predestined to become cholinergic; in that case the conditioning factor would enhance the survival and growth of the cholinergic population while diminishing that of the adrenergic population. This hypothesis is unlikely, however, since conditioned medium has no effect either on the survival or growth of cultured neurons. A second possibility is that the conditioned medium induces the expression of cholinergic properties in a predetermined cholinergic population that otherwise survives but does not express any transmitter metabolism. This hypothesis was also ruled out by the finding that in the absence of conditioned medium virtually no neurons were "silent" with respect to transmitter synthesis.

A third explanation for the effect of conditioned medium is the most consistent with our observa-

Figure 60 CULTURED NEURON obtained from the sympathetic ganglion of a newborn rat sprouts fine branching extensions when incubated in the presence of nerve-growth factor (NGF). The micrographs show the cell after 240 minutes of incubation (*top left*), 300 minutes (*top right*) and 500 minutes (*bottom*). The extensions grow continuously and eventually form a meshwork over the surface of the culture dish. They may also form synapses with other neurons or with cultured muscle cells. (Micrograph by D. Bray of Medical Research Council Cell Biophysics Unit, London.)

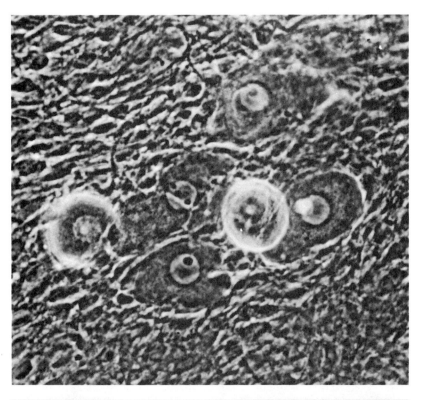

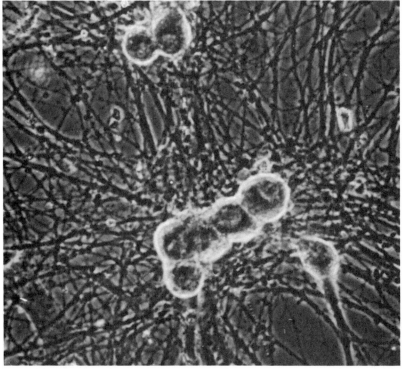

Figure 61 IMMATURE NEU-RONS from sympathetic ganglia of a newborn rat. In standard medium the non-neuronal supporting cells of the ganglion survive and divide, forming a continuous layer around and beneath the neurons (*top*). Cultures that contain only neurons (*bottom*) can be prepared by growing ganglionic cells in a medium in which neurons survive but non-neuronal cells do not. One such medium contains cytosine arabinoside, which is toxic when incorporated into the nucleic acid molecules of the dividing non-neuronal cells but does not affect the neurons, which merely grow larger.

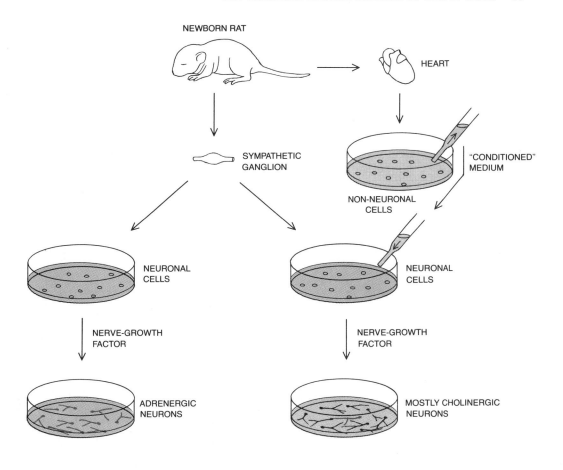

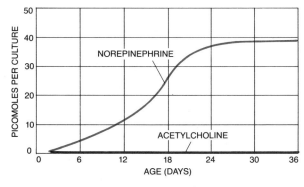

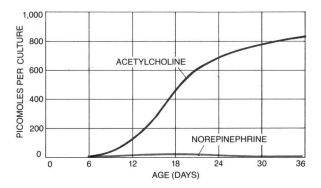

Figure 62 EFFECT OF CULTURE ENVIRONMENT. If immature neurons from the sympathetic ganglia of newborn rats are grown in pure cultures, nearly all manufacture and secrete norepinephrine. If the immature neurons are cultured together with non-neuronal cells, or if they are treated with culture medium that has been incubated with non-neuronal cells, a large majority of the neurons will manufacture and secrete acetylcholine. In the absence of conditioned medium (*left graph*) the ability to make norepinephrine rises over three weeks and the ability to make acetylcholine remains negligible. In sister cultures grown in 62 percent conditioned medium (*right graph*) the ability to make norepinephrine first rises then declines as ability to make acetylcholine rises.

tions. According to this hypothesis the neurons that express adrenergic properties at the outset are still "plastic" with respect to neurotransmitter choice for a considerable period after birth and can become cholinergic under the influence of conditioned medium. This concept implies that the active ingredient of conditioned medium determines the choice of transmitter and the type of synapses made by a sympathetic neuron without affecting whether the neuron survives or how extensive its axon and dendrites are.

The reciprocity in the expression of adrenergic and cholinergic functions can be ascribed to a "competition" of some kind within each neuron between the prenatal instruction to become adrenergic and the new instruction to become cholinergic. If such a competition exists, one may ask if an individual neuron can express both transmitter systems simultaneously, at least for a short period. We attempted to answer the question by growing single neurons on small beds of heart-muscle cells from a newborn rat for about two weeks. The cells were

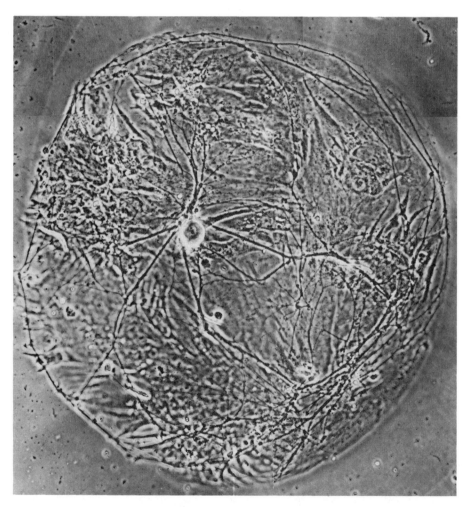

Figure 63 SINGLE NEURON (*center*) **extends its branches over a background layer of heart cells in a microculture system. The transmitter secreted by the neuron can be identified by its effect on the cardiac muscle cells, which contract spontaneously and rhythmically in culture. Once the neuron is attached, its threadlike extensions form syn-aptic connections with some cardiac muscle cells. The neurotransmitter secreted at the synapses is either acetylcholine, which slows the beating of the cells, or norepinephrine, which accelerates it, and at a certain stage in differentiation some neurons secrete both.**

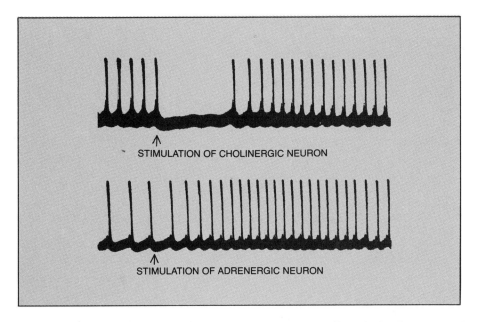

STIMULATION OF CHOLINERGIC NEURON

STIMULATION OF ADRENERGIC NEURON

Figure 64 FREQUENCY OF CONTRACTION of the cardiac muscle cells in a single neuron reveals the identity of the neurotransmitter secreted by that neuron. A microelectrode inserted into the neuron stimulates the release of transmitter as a second microelectrode in an innervated muscle cell monitors the cell's contractions. Trace at the **top shows the effect of stimulating a cholinergic neuron: spontaneous contractions of the muscle cell cease temporarily. Bottom trace shows effect of stimulating an adrenergic neuron: contraction frequency of the innervated cell increases.**

plated onto tiny disks of collagen about .5 millimeter in diameter to which they attach preferentially. One such disk is shown in Figure 63. The neuron and an adjacent heart cell in such microcultures were impaled with microelectrodes to monitor their electrical activity; in that way the transmitter choice of the neuron could be assayed by triggering the release of the transmitter and observing its effect on the heart cells, which "beat" spontaneously and rhythmically in culture. Unlike the cultured sympathetic neurons, the heart cells possess both cholinergic receptors and electrically active adrenergic receptors; thus a slowing or stopping of the beating indicates the secretion of acetylcholine, whereas an increased frequency of the beating indicates the secretion of norepinephrine. Further evidence for the identity of the transmitter can be obtained by observing the effects of certain drugs that compete specifically with the natural transmitter for binding to the receptors on the heart cells. For example, atropine blocks cardiac acetylcholine receptors, whereas propranolol blocks cardiac norepinephrine receptors.

Working with this technique we have identified three types of neurons in the two-week-old microcultures. The first type is adrenergic: it excites the heart cells and the effect is blocked by propranolol. The second type is cholinergic: it inhibits the heart cells and the effect is blocked by atropine. The third type of neuron exhibits both cholinergic and adrenergic activity: stimulation of the neuron inhibits the heart with an atropine-sensitive mechanism and then speeds up the heart with a propranolol-sensitive mechanism. Since only one neuron is present in each microculture, it is clear that the same cell mediates both effects. When the microcultures are examined with the electron microscope, numerous dense-core synaptic vesicles are seen in the adrenergic neurons, clear vesicles are seen in the cholinergic neurons and a few dense-core vesicles combined with a large majority of clear vesicles are seen in the dual-function cells. An obvious advantage of studying cultures that contain only one neuron is that it is possible to make an unambiguous correlation between the structure and function of the cell.

These findings establish that a single neuron can express both transmitter systems simultaneously at an immature stage. Dual function may seem to be a

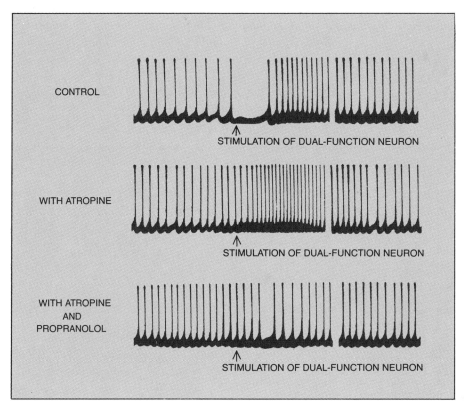

Figure 65 DUAL-FUNCTION NEURON. In the trace at top stimulation of the neuron causes a cessation of the beating of the innervated cardiac muscle cells (mediated by acetylcholine) then a resumption of beating at an enhanced rate (mediated by norepinephrine). In the lower two traces drugs that specifically block either cholinergic or adrener- **gic transmission have been added to culture medium to verify dual function. With atropine the inhibition is removed but the excitation remains intact. By adding propranolol both the excitatory and inhibitory effects of the neuron are blocked.**

novel concept, but developing neurons have not previously been investigated in ways that might reveal this behavior. In retrospect dual function is a logical intermediate step in the conversion of an adrenergic neuron to a cholinergic neuron under the influence of conditioned medium. Even if there is no temporal overlap between the synthesis of enzymes and other components involved in manufacture and release of the two neurotransmitters, it is reasonable to assume that the enzymes and synaptic vesicles involved in adrenergic transmission would continue to function for a while after their synthesis had ceased. The precise duration of the dual-function state is not yet known.

After about four weeks the single neurons in microculture have grown so large that biochemical assays can be made on them. The cells are

incubated in a mixture of radioactive tyrosine and choline for eight to 12 hours; then the amount of norepinephrine and acetylcholine that have been synthesized from these precursor molecules is determined. In the absence of conditioned medium virtually all the neurons make detectable quantities only of norepinephrine. In the presence of heart cells, however, a substantial majority of the neurons make only acetylcholine. Under no circumstances is there a significant number of "silent" or dual-function neurons after four weeks in culture.

These findings indicate that most neurons are adrenergic at the time they are put into culture but are susceptible to a "flip-flop" control mechanism that determines their ultimate choice of transmitter. The duration of the transition period during which dual function may be expressed is not known, but by four or five weeks after birth virtually all the neurons have differentiated into a state in which only one transmitter system is expressed to a significant degree. We are currently following the status of single neurons over a period of time by intermittently testing their effects on heart cells. In this way we hope to observe the transition from adrenergic to cholinergic behavior directly and to determine its time course.

When in the life of the culture are the neurons most sensitive to the action of conditioned medium, and how reversible are its effects? To answer these questions conditioned medium was added to cultures of sympathetic neurons for a 10-day "pulse" at various stages of cell maturity. We found that the responsiveness of the cells to the pulse of conditioned medium declined rapidly with the increasing age of the cells, reaching a very low level when the pulse was applied between days 40 and 50. Caryl Hill and Ian Hendry of the Australian National University and C. David Ross, Mary Johnson and Bunge of the Washington University School of Medicine obtained similar results in intact animals. When small pieces of sympathetic ganglia were taken from rats of various ages and placed in culture for a standard period, the expression of cholinergic function declined progressively with increasing age of the animal from which the explant was taken, reaching a minimum in the ganglia of adult rats.

One of the most intriguing aspects of the influence of non-neuronal cells on the choice of neurotransmitter is the distribution of effectiveness among the various non-neuronal cells of the body. If this property were properly localized, it might act as a specific determinant of transmitter choice. To investigate the matter we studied the effect of various tissues from the newborn rat on transmitter choice. All the non-neuronal cells were able to induce cholinergic function, but there were clear quantitative differences in effectiveness: cells from skeletal muscle were most effective, cells from the heart were intermediate and cells from the liver were least effective. A conspicuous feature of this order was its relation to the amount of cholinergic innervation received by the target tissue: skeletal muscle fibers receive only cholinergic input, heart-muscle cells a mixture of cholinergic and adrenergic input, and liver cells, when they are innervated at all, only adrenergic input. This finding suggested that during development target cells release chemical factors that influence the transmitter metabolism of the neurons that innervate them.

Other observations did not, however, appear to be encompassed by this simple hypothesis. Several types of cells that are effective medium conditioners are not normally innervated, in the sense

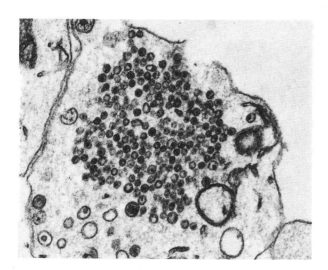

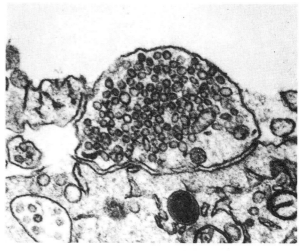

Figure 66 SYNAPTIC VARICOSITIES along the axons of cultured cholinergic or adrenergic neurons display characteristic differences in their fine structure. The molecules of neurotransmitter are stored in synaptic vesicles. When the varicosities of adrenergic neurons are stained with per-manganate and examined in the electron microscope, they contain synaptic vesicles with small, electron-dense cores (*left*). The varicosities of cholinergic neurons have vesicles with clear interiors (*right*). (Micrographs by S. C. Landis of Harvard Medical School.)

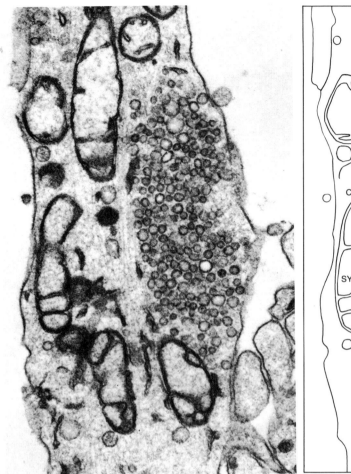

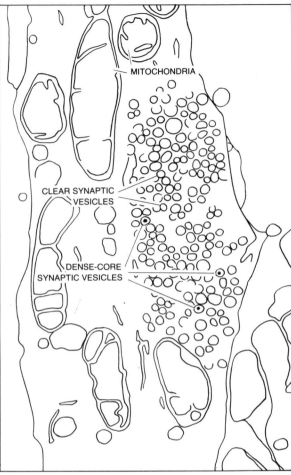

MITOCHONDRIA

CLEAR SYNAPTIC VESICLES

DENSE-CORE SYNAPTIC VESICLES

Figure 67 DUAL-FUNCTION VARICOSITY contains a few dense-core vesicles characteristic of an adrenergic neuron (*see map*) with a large majority of clear vesicles characteristic of a cholinergic neuron. Thus the fine structure of the varicosity is correlated with its combined inhibitory and excitatory effects. The dual-function state is thought to be a transient phase during the conversion of an adrenergic neuron to a cholinergic one under influence of conditioned medium. (Micrograph by S. C. Landis.)

of receiving synapses. Among these cells are fibroblasts (connective-tissue cells), a line of glial tumor cells serially propagated in culture (glial cells are the supporting cells of neurons in the brain and spinal cord) and the non-neuronal cells in sympathetic ganglia. The ability of ganglionic non-neuronal cells to induce cholinergic differentiation seemed particularly paradoxical. During the first three weeks after birth the non-neuronal cells in the ganglion surround each neuron closely, yet most of the neurons in the intact ganglia end up adrenergic. Why is it that non-neuronal cells or conditioned medium can cause almost all sympathetic neurons to become cholinergic in culture, yet in the body only a few sympathetic neurons become cholinergic even in

the presence of an abundance of non-neuronal cells?

This apparent paradox indicated that additional variables were involved in the choice of transmitter. The sympathetic neurons in the body were exposed to the cholinergic signal provided by the non-neuronal cells, yet most of them were prevented from responding to the signal by some factor that was missing from the culture medium. One possible candidate for this factor was NGF, since it is critical for the survival and growth of adrenergic sympathetic neurons both in the intact animal and in culture. Moreover, when neuronal cultures are exposed to high concentrations of NGF, there is an increase in the manufacture of specifically adrenergic components, such as norepinephrine, relative to the manufacture of nonspecific cell components such as protein and lipid. It turns out, however, that NGF has the same potentiating effect on cholinergic differentiation. Thus with respect to transmitter production NGF is permissive rather than instructive: it stimulates the growth and differentiation of immature sympathetic neurons along either the adrenergic path or the cholinergic one but does not influence which path is taken. In contrast to NGF the cholinergic factor secreted by non-neuronal cells

does not affect neuronal survival or growth but does instruct the neurons with respect to neurotransmitter choice.

Another candidate for the factor in the intact animal that prevented the majority of sympathetic neurons from becoming cholinergic was the normal excitatory input from the central neurons, which were absent from our cultures. Ira Black, Hendry and Leslie Iversen at the Medical Research Council Laboratory of Molecular Biology in Cambridge, England, had found that if the spinal input to the

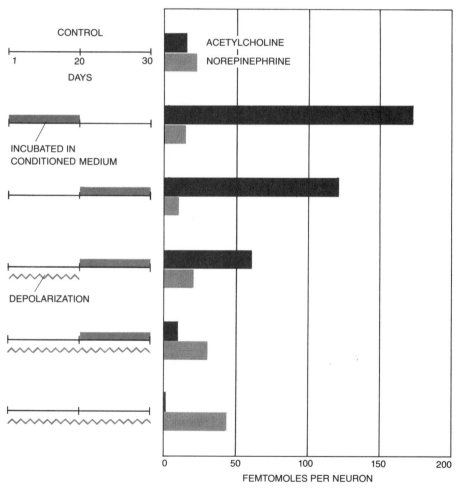

Figure 68 ELECTRICAL ACTIVITY of sympathetic neurons reduce their ability to become cholinergic when they are exposed to conditioned medium. The excitatory influence of spinal neurons can be mimicked in cell culture by treating the sympathetic neurons with potassium ion, which depolarizes them. Potassium or conditioned medium was added on days 0 or 20, and each transmitter manufactured was assayed on day 30. Depolarization largely blocked the effect of conditioned medium. The minority of neurons in the intact sympathetic ganglion that end up cholinergic may not become electrically active until they undergo cholinergic induction by non-neuronal cells.

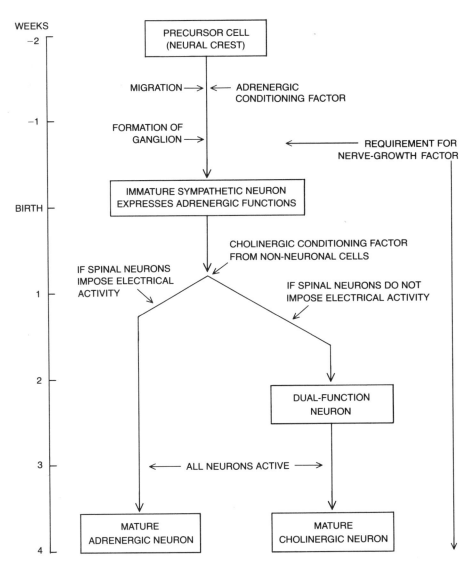

WEEKS

−2 ─ PRECURSOR CELL
(NEURAL CREST)

MIGRATION → ← ADRENERGIC
CONDITIONING FACTOR

−1 ─ FORMATION OF
GANGLION →

← REQUIREMENT FOR
NERVE-GROWTH FACTOR

BIRTH ─ IMMATURE SYMPATHETIC NEURON
EXPRESSES ADRENERGIC FUNCTIONS

CHOLINERGIC CONDITIONING FACTOR
FROM NON-NEURONAL CELLS

IF SPINAL NEURONS
IMPOSE ELECTRICAL
ACTIVITY

IF SPINAL NEURONS DO NOT
IMPOSE ELECTRICAL ACTIVITY

1 ─

2 ─ DUAL-FUNCTION
NEURON

3 ─ ← ALL NEURONS ACTIVE →

MATURE
ADRENERGIC NEURON

MATURE
CHOLINERGIC NEURON

4 ─

Figure 69 FLOW CHART represents a hypothesis about the developmental steps involved in the chemical differentiation of a sympathetic neuron. According to the hypothesis the environmental influences that affect the cell's choice of neurotransmitter are exerted both by non-neuronal cells (which release developmental factors) and by other neurons (whose electrical activity modifies the neuron's response to the factors). Time axis is approximate. Since development of the neurons is not yet synchronized, they would traverse the pathways at somewhat different times.

sympathetic ganglia of young mice is cut, further development of the adrenergic metabolism is reduced. These observations raised the possibility that electrical activity imposed on the ganglionic neurons during the first week after birth plays a role in determining the choice of transmitter. Although the innervating central neurons are not present in the cell culture, we were able to mimic their excitatory effect on the ganglionic neurons (in which the membrane of the neuron is depolarized, that is, the voltage across the membrane is reversed). This was done by raising the potassium concentration of the medium, by adding the drug veratridine, which causes an influx of sodium ions into the neurons, or by stimulating the cells electrically once per second for many days.

When mass neuronal cultures were depolarized either in the presence of conditioned medium or for seven to 10 days before the addition of conditioned medium, the neurons remained primarily adrenergic. Indeed, depolarization depressed the ratio of acetylcholine synthesis to norepinephrine synthesis as much as 300-fold compared with cultures that simply received conditioned medium. These changes occurred without a significant alteration in the survival of neurons, suggesting that the neurons, which would have become cholinergic in response to conditioned medium, now remained adrenergic. It was as if the depolarization of the sympathetic neurons stabilized their prenatal instruction to become adrenergic and curtailed their plasticity with respect to transmitter choice.

Electrical activity is accompanied by the entry of calcium ions into neurons. Because the entry of calcium ions is important in controlling the secretion of neurotransmitters and probably other cellular functions, the question arose whether the effects of depolarization on transmitter choice could be diminished by preventing the influx of calcium. This was done by raising the concentration of magnesium ions in the medium or by adding the drug D600, which selectively blocks the movement of calcium ions across the cell membrane. Indeed, when calcium entry was blocked, depolarization no longer prevented the induction of cholinergic properties by conditioned medium. Thus the effect of depolarization in blocking the effect of conditioned medium on transmitter choice appears to be mediated through calcium ions, although the precise mechanism is not yet understood.

These observations raise the possibility that in the intact ganglia the majority of neurons are preserved in their prenatal adrenergic condition by electrical input from the spinal cord that begins during the first week after birth. A corollary hypothesis is that the neurons in the ganglia that are destined to become cholinergic (those that innervate certain blood vessels and sweat glands) acquire their electrical input only after they have been influenced by the non-neuronal cells. Inherent in such a mechanism is an interesting possibility. Perhaps the selective formation of synapses between the central neurons and the ganglionic neurons not only establishes the circuitry of the autonomic pathways but also determines the choice of transmitter that is appropriate to the circuitry. This concept emphasizes the potential importance of neuronal activity in the chemical differentiation of the nervous system.

The experiments described in this article leave little doubt that developing sympathetic neurons are at least transiently plastic with respect to their choice of transmitter. A similar conclusion has recently been reached by Nicole Le Douarin and her colleagues at the Institute of Embryology at No-

gentsur-Marne in France, who are doing ingenious transplantation experiments in bird embryos. They find that the decision of immature neurons to become adrenergic or cholinergic can be altered if the cells are transplanted to new sites in the embryo. For example, a precursor population that normally gives rise to cholinergic neurons will yield adrenergic neurons if it is transplanted to a region where adrenergic neurons normally arise. In sum, both in culture and in intact embryos, this important neuronal decision is not entirely preprogrammed but can be influenced by other cells, including neurons and non-neuronal cells.

We have discussed here the control of just one decision in the development of a single class of nerve cells. The development of the intricate synaptic network of the adult nervous system presumably involves almost innumerable decisions, many of which also depend on cellular interactions. Disentangling these interactions is likely to require a combination of research approaches, including the study of development in the embryo and in simplified and controlled culture environments. Ultimately one would like to be able to specify everything that must be added to a culture dish to cause an embryonic neuron to display its entire range of behavior from the time cell division ceases to senescence.

POSTSCRIPT

Much progress has been made in this field (see work by Patterson, 1987), but the information in this chapter remains the foundation for much of the current efforts. Perhaps the most exciting recent finding is that the changes in phenotype that Drs. Patterson, Potter and Furshpan observed in vitro have been found to represent stages of normal development in vivo. In addition, the molecular signals that control changes in transmitter and vesicle phenotype during development have been identified. For example, in superior cervical ganglion cells and in chromaffin cells corticosteroids and nerve growth factor (NGF) play both permissive and instructive roles (Doupe, Patterson and Landis, 1985). The voltage-dependent entry of calcium ions is a signal in some cells in culture, probably reflecting their requirement for innervation in vivo (Gallo et al., 1987 and Liles and Nathanson, 1987). In addition to the classical neurotransmitters, the peptide phenotype can be altered in sympathetic neurons in culture (Kessler, 1985).

GABAergic Neurons

Nerve cells not only excite their neighbors but also inhibit them. Such inhibitory activity—often mediated by an amino acid known as GABA—helps to shape the neural networks that underlie all behavior.

. . .

David I. Gottlieb

February, 1988

One usually conceives of the activity of the nervous system as a pattern of excitations. Sensory stimuli are converted into impulses that are relayed from nerve cell to nerve cell before ultimately being converted into responses. By and large this picture is an appropriate one. Yet there is an entire class of operations in the nervous system that are not excitations at all but inhibitions, and these operations are mediated by a special class of inhibitory neurons (nerve cells). Rather than exciting its target cell, the firing of an inhibitory neuron damps the target's firing or eliminates it altogether. The constraining action is accomplished by the release of specific molecules called inhibitory transmitters. Among the most prevalent of them is a simple amino acid called gamma-aminobutyric acid, or GABA; neurons that secrete GABA are referred to by neurobiologists as GABAergic.

GABA was established as an inhibitory neurotransmitter by a long line of experiments begun in the 1950's. Within the past five years the techniques of molecular biology have made great new strides possible. By means of those techniques much has been learned about GABA, about the enzyme that makes it

and about the receptor to which it binds. At the same time the function of inhibitory neural networks is becoming clearer. Not only do such circuits act as brakes on the entire nervous system—preventing a runaway spree of neural firing—but also they help to "tune" the specific responsiveness of the excitatory networks that convey and interpret information about the external world. Indeed, as more is understood about inhibitory networks, they seem increasingly to be equal partners with the excitatory circuitry that generally dominates one's thinking about the activity of the nervous system.

In the investigation of the nervous system most of the attention was initially concentrated on the excitatory pathways. By the 1940's a considerable amount was known about how the excitatory impulse is generated and conveyed from neuron to neuron. An excitatory signal travels along a neuron as a minute electrical change. Ordinarily the inside of a neuron has a net negative electric potential with respect to the outside of the cell; the difference is maintained by pumps and channels that distribute electrically charged ions (such as those of sodium, potassium and chlorine) differently on the inside and outside of the cell. As the electrical impulse, or "action potential," passes along the neuron, channels open and close, allowing ions to flow, and the inside of the cell briefly becomes positive with respect to the outside before returning to the resting level.

The action potential travels away from the body of the cell along an axon (the type of fiber that sends nerve signals). At the end of the axon it reaches the synaptic terminal, a bulbous structure forming the "near" side of the synapse, or gap, between nerve cells. The arrival of the action potential causes a rapid discharge of neurotransmitter from the terminal into the synaptic cleft. The transmitter diffuses across the synapse and binds to receptor molecules on a dendrite (receiving fiber) of the second neuron. The interaction of transmitter and receptor elicits a new electrical signal in the dendrite. Synapses are so well adapted to their function that this complex process takes place in about a thousandth of a second.

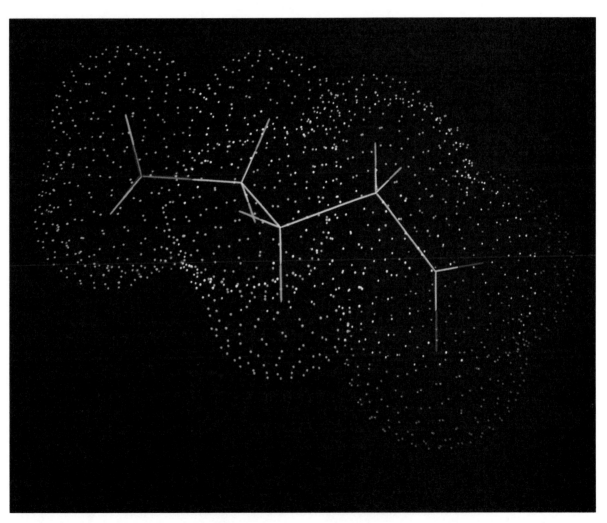

Figure 70 GAMMA-AMINOBUTRYIC ACID (GABA) is an amino acid and an inhibitory neurotransmitter. This computer image shows the atomic structure of GABA (*lines*) and the distribution of the surrounding electric charge (*clouds of dots*). Yellow-white corresponds to carbon, blue-green to hydrogen, blue to nitrogen and red to oxygen. (Image by G. R. Marshall of the Washington University School of Medicine.)

By the 1950's, however, it had become clear that not all synapses work this way: many of them block the activity of the postsynaptic neuron. It was reasonable to assume that specialized transmitters are responsible for the inhibitory effect. Quickly evidence began to accumulate suggesting that GABA is one such molecule. In the early 1950's Eugene Roberts of Washington University in St. Louis, Jorge Awapara of the University of Texas and Sidney Udenfriend of the National Heart Institute independently discovered that GABA is present in high concentrations in mammalian brain tissue. The amino acid was undetectable in other organs, which implied that it has a specific role in the central nervous system. The complexity of the mammalian brain, however, made it difficult to specify what that role might be.

Fortunately a workable model was soon provided by simpler organisms: the crustaceans. The muscle fibers of lobsters and crayfish receive three different neural inputs. Excitatory axons extend from the central ganglia (the nodes of neural tissue along the midline of the body that serve as switching points for the nervous system) to the muscle fibers; activation of the excitatory neurons causes the muscle to contract. A second type of neuron runs from the muscle fiber to the central ganglia. Called the stretch-receptor neuron, it conveys information about muscle length to the central nodes. Finally, there are inhibitory axons that are connected to both the muscle fibers and the stretch-receptor cells. When the inhibitory neurons fire, they suppress the activity of the muscle and the stretch receptors.

Several lines of evidence demonstrate conclusively that GABA is the inhibitory neurotransmitter of this system. Ernst Florey of McGill University showed that GABA, applied to a preparation of isolated muscle fiber and neurons, suppresses the discharge of the stretch receptor; others showed that GABA does the same for muscle fibers. A plant alkaloid called picrotoxin, which blocks the action of GABA, also blocks the action of the inhibitory axons specifically and reversibly. What is more, both GABA and the enzyme that makes it—glutamic acid decarboxylase (GAD)—are found in the inhibitory axons but not in the excitatory ones. The distribution of the enzyme was uncovered by a team from the Harvard Medical School that was led by Stephen W. Kuffler and Edward A. Kramt and also included J. Dudel, David D. Potter and Zach Hall.

The crowning touch was then provided by the Harvard investigators, who dissected the crustacean

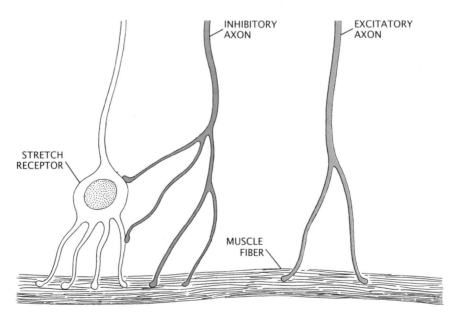

Figure 71 SIMPLE EXPERIMENTAL SYSTEM consisting of nerve and muscle fibers from a crustacean provided the basis for proving that GABA is an inhibitory transmitter. The excitatory axon, coming from the main nerve bundles near the midline of the body, causes the muscle fiber to contract. The stretch receptor conveys information about the contractional state of the muscle. The inhibitory axon blocks muscular contraction and the firing of the stretch receptor.

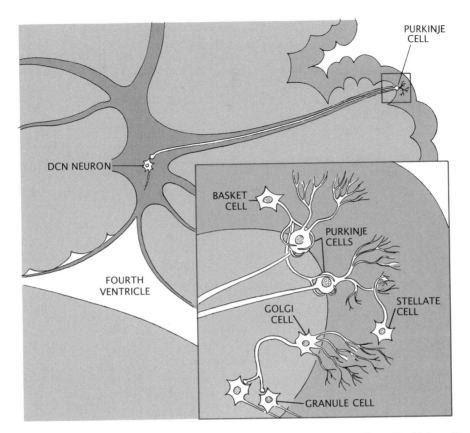

Figure 72 CORTEX OF CEREBELLUM (shown in cross section) exercises its effects on other brain structures solely by means of inhibitory neurons. The output of the cerebellum is carried by neurons coming from the deep cerebellar nuclei (DCN). All the axons extending from the cortex to the DCN are derived from Purkinje cells, inhibitory neurons whose transmitter is GABA. The Purkinje cells are part of a complex network of neurons with both excitatory and inhibitory inputs (*inset*).

neuromuscular preparation free of surrounding tissue and placed it in a saline bath. Stimulation of the inhibitory axons, but not the excitatory ones, caused the release of GABA into the bath. Taken together, these results clearly showed that GABA is the inhibitory transmitter in the crustacean system. The wideranging series of experiments carried out by the Harvard workers served as an often emulated model for establishing the nature of the transmitter at other synapses, and by the 1960's the focus of the attack had shifted back to the mammalian brain.

A wealth of evidence from many areas of the brain confirms that GABA is an inhibitory transmitter in the brains of all mammals, human beings included. One of the areas where GABAergic neurons have been best studied is the cortex (outer layer) of the cerebellum. The cerebellar cortex is responsible

for the smooth coordination of muscular activity, a job it carries out by influencing neurons in various higher-brain structures. Of the neurons in the cerebellar cortex only the one called the Purkinje cell has an axon that leaves that structure: the Purkinje cell axons terminate in structures called the deep cerebellar nuclei (DCN) that lie underneath the cortex. As a result of this arrangement the cortex can influence other brain structures only through the action of Purkinje cells.

In the early 1960's Masao Ito of the University of Tokyo and his colleagues made a surprising discovery. They found that stimulating the Purkinje cells caused the rate of firing of the neurons in the DCN to decrease rather than increase. Their conclusion was that the Purkinje cells' action is inhibitory. Since the Purkinje cells provide the sole route from the cerebellar cortex to the underlying nuclei, it follows that the cortex exercises all its effect on the rest of the brain through inhibition.

It was not long before it was found that the transmitter that mediates the inhibitory effect is GABA. The evidence followed the lines that had been established in the crustacean work. When GABA is applied to the cells of the DCN, their firing is blocked. Agents such as picrotoxin and another substance called bicuculline, which block the effect of GABA, also block activity in the synapses made by Purkinje cells. The Purkinje cells contain high levels of GAD and GABA. Demonstrating that GABA is released when Purkinje cells fire was the most difficult task, but K. Obata and K. Takeda of Tokyo Medical University found an elegant way to measure the release of transmitter into the fourth ventricle (the large, fluid-filled cavity above which the DCN lie). They showed that the firing of Purkinje cells is indeed accompanied by the release of GABA.

Once it had been clearly demonstrated that GABA is an inhibitory transmitter in the mammalian brain, work progressed rapidly, yielding a picture of the "typical" GABAergic neuron. GABAergic neurons contain high concentrations of the synthesizing enzyme GAD. The enzyme is found throughout the cell, but it is particularly concentrated in the presynaptic terminal. Within the terminal are many vesicles, and it is thought that the stored GABA is released from the vesicles, although firm evidence is still lacking on this point. In addition, the outer membrane of the terminal incorporates molecular pumps that help to clear the synapse of GABA, preparing the synapse for the next firing (see Figure 74).

To have its effect, GABA not only must be released but also must be bound on the postsynaptic side of the synapse by receptors: molecules specific for that purpose embedded in the outer membrane of the postsynaptic cell. In the case of GABA there are two such receptors, designated GABA$_A$ and GABA$_B$. Each receptor binds GABA and then produces a change in ion permeability. In the case of the A receptor the permeability of the membrane to chloride ion is increased; in the case of the B receptor it is the potassium permeability that increases. In both instances the effect is the same: the potential difference between the inside and the outside of the postsynaptic cell increases, and so the cell becomes less likely to fire.

GABAergic neurons are widespread in the central nervous system. Almost every major division of the brain and spinal cord includes some of them. In many regions they make up an appreciable minority of all neurons: between 20 and 40 percent. Remarkably, in some regions these inhibitory neurons actually make up the majority of all the nerve cells that are present.

On the basis of their anatomical form GABAergic neurons have been divided into three groups. Type I neurons have many processes, or extensions, but the processes are not clearly divided into dendrites and axons, as is the case for most nerve cells. Instead each process is both a sender and a receiver of messages. An example is provided by the granule cells of the olfactory bulb, which outnumber all other neurons there and inhibit specific neighboring cells.

In Type II and Type III neurons, on the other hand, dendrites and axons are clearly distinguished. All Type II cells send messages to other neurons within the adjacent gray matter of the brain (which consists of nerve bodies, nerve fibers and supportive tissue), but they can vary widely in the number of cells with which they make contact. For example, the basket cell (a Type II neuron in the cerebellum) generally synapses with about six Purkinje cells; its neighbor, the Golgi cell, however, may make connections with up to 10,000 of its target cells. Type III neurons are called projection neurons because their axons leave the gray matter and enter the white matter (which consists largely of nerve-fiber bundles), thereby serving to inhibit neurons in distant brain structures.

It is not yet clear how the anatomical form of each GABAergic neuron is correlated with its function, and the problem is under active investigation. In the meantime a considerable amount has been learned at the molecular level about how GABAergic synapses operate. Such knowledge has been gleaned partly at the intersection of pharmacology and molecular biology. As it happens, the pharmacological insights were gained first. The 1960's was the decade when the benzodiazepines came into widespread use. This class of chemicals, whose best-known member is marketed under the name Valium, is prescribed to relieve anxiety, pain and muscle spasms, to induce sleep and for acute (but not chronic) control of epilepsy.

Quite early, Erminio Costa of the National Institute of Mental Health showed that the benzodiazepines can have such varied effects because they potentiate (augment) the action of GABA. Further work by Gerald D. Fischbach, Dennis W. Choi

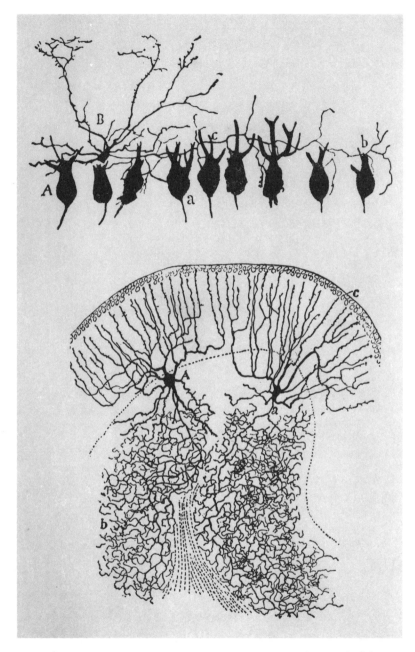

Figure 73 INHIBITORY NEURONS have a broad range of anatomical forms. Drawings by the 19th-century neuroanatomist Santiago Ramón y Cajal depict neurons that are now known to be inhibitory. The upper panel shows a basket cell (*B*) with a row of Purkinje cells (*A*). The lower panel shows a pair of Golgi cells; the tangled masses below the cell bodies are the axons.

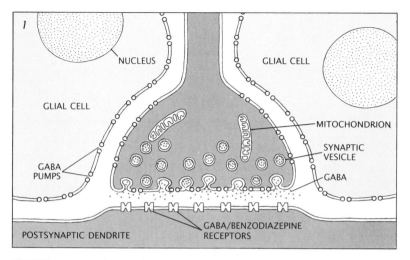

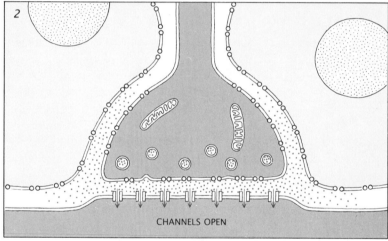

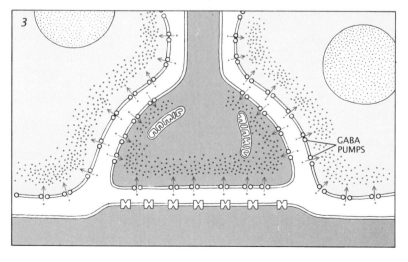

Figure 74 SYNAPTIC TRANS-MITTER must be cleared from the extracellular space so that the synapse may convey the next signal. This is done by pumps in the membrane of the axon and surrounding glial cells. On being released by vesicles (*1*), GABA crosses the synapse and binds to specific receptor molecules in the membrane of the postsynaptic dendrite (*2*). The binding changes the membrane's permeability to such ions as chloride and potassium. Molecular pumps then quickly begin removing GABA from the synapse (*3*).

and David H. Farb of the Harvard Medical School and Jeffery L. Barker and Robert Macdonald of the National Institute of Mental Health demonstrated that the augmentation takes place at the level of the GABA receptor. As I have described above, one type of GABA receptor controls chloride permeability. The Harvard and NIMH groups showed that the benzodiazepines lower the concentration of GABA needed to increase chloride permeability. Significantly, the drugs do not affect permeability when they are administered alone: they can only intensify the effect of the normal transmitter. It is now known that the benzodiazepines bind to the GABA receptor at a site different from the site where GABA binds, but their precise mechanism is not understood.

In the 1980's, studies of GABAergic neurons have expanded to include molecular biology along with pharmacology. Even in molecular-biological studies, however, the benzodiazepines provided a crucial foothold, as I shall describe.

Until recently students of the central nervous system felt as if they were to some extent excluded from the unfolding drama of molecular biology. The great complexity of the mammalian brain made neurobiologists despair of learning anything by the rapidly advancing methods of molecular genetics. In the past few years, however, it has become possible to analyze key brain genes and proteins with the full power of molecular biology. That power has been applied to both GAD, the enzyme that makes GABA, and the GABA receptor, with intriguing results.

The new techniques have made it possible to achieve results much more quickly than they could possibly have been achieved with the older methods of classical protein chemistry. The older methods were beset with difficulty, mainly because both GAD and the GABA receptor are present in very small quantities in the brain and are difficult to separate from the multitude of other brain proteins. In their pioneering studies on the structure of GAD, Roberts and Jan-Yen Wu of the City of Hope Medical Center were forced to liquefy more than 9,000 mouse brains to obtain enough of the enzyme to perform analytical studies. Clearly, under such conditions the work on GAD would have progressed slowly.

One of the most effective tools in the kit of molecular biology is the monoclonal antibody: an antibody that binds specifically and exclusively to a single protein. With such an antibody in hand one can separate a protein from its environment, no matter how complex that environment is. Recently my colleagues Yen-Chung Chang and James Schwob and I succeeded in preparing a monoclonal antibody to GAD. Having such a monoclonal antibody makes it possible to purify the enzyme rapidly and in high yield, which has enabled us to work out part of the amino acid sequence of the enzyme and further analyze its molecular composition.

An even more detailed look at GAD has been obtained by means of another of the ingenious tools of the new molecular biology: the complementary DNA (cDNA) clone. Such a DNA clone is called complementary because it matches the messenger RNA (mRNA) for a particular protein, in this case the enzyme GAD. Because the cDNA carries the genetic information that specifies the string of amino acids in the protein, analysis of the clone yields the complete sequence of amino acids, a most valuable piece of information. Obtaining the clone, however, is no small feat. In this case the job was done by Daniel L. Kaufman and Allan J. Tobin of the University of California at Los Angeles.

Kaufman and Tobin first prepared a cDNA "library" from the brain of a cat. The library includes cDNA's that are complementary to all species of messenger RNA found in the cat's brain. The next step was to select, from among all the DNA's in the library, the one corresponding to the desired enzyme. In order to do so, the library was inserted into a simple virus called a phage that infects bacteria; one small piece of the library was put into each phage. Once inside the bacterium, the DNA carried by the phage is expressed, or used to make protein. When that happens, antibodies to GAD can be used to pick out the bacteria carrying the DNA for the enzyme. Tobin's group sequenced the clone and deduced the entire amino acid sequence of GAD.

The GABA receptor is an even more elusive protein than the enzyme that makes GABA: it accounts for only one part in 50,000 of all brain protein. Yet a series of experiments that entailed a crucial exploitation of the benzodiazepines has made it possible to understand the basic structure of the receptor.

The GABA receptor is an integral membrane protein: it extends through the bilayered outer membrane of the postsynaptic neuron. Richard W. Olsen of the University of California at Los Angeles first showed that the intact and functional receptor could be separated from the membrane by means of detergents. Building on Olsen's work, Eric A. Barnard of the U.K. Medical Research Council's Molecular Neurobiology Unit and Hans Möhler of the

Roche Company in Switzerland have been able to separate the receptor from the mass of other proteins embedded in the membrane. After being released from the membrane with detergent, the proteins were passed through a column packed with minute beads to which benzodiazepine molecules were bound. The benzodiazepines hooked the passing GABA receptors, which were then stripped from the column so that they could be analyzed chemically.

The benzodiazepines, it should be noted, bind only to the GABA$_A$ receptor. Hence the receptor molecule removed from the column as the A-type receptor, which, as I mentioned, affects the permeability of the membrane to chloride ions. The analysis carried out by the British and Swiss groups showed that the GABA$_A$ receptor consists of two conjoined subunits, one of about 55,000 daltons and the other of about 50,000 daltons. (A dalton is a measure of molecular weight equal to the weight of a single atom of hydrogen.) What is more, having the purified receptor molecule made it possible to prepare monoclonal antibodies and take other steps that laid the groundwork for cloning the receptor gene.

Just last July, Barnard's group reported that they had cloned the genes for the GABA$_A$ receptor. Several significant results followed from their breakthrough. First, as in the case of GAD, the genes yielded the complete amino acid sequence of the paired receptor subunits. Knowledge of the sequence provided the basis for formulating a model of the receptor's geometry and position in the membrane. The structure reported by Barnard's group in their paper includes a set of eight helical regions spanning the membrane (four per subunit) connected by linear stretches. The helical units probably form the channel through which the chloride ions pass.

Not content with that substantial advance, Barnard and his co-workers took two further steps. The first was to inject mRNA's corresponding to the receptor genes into oocytes (eggs) from a frog of the genus *Xenopus*. In the egg the RNA's made their way to ribosomes, where they were translated into receptor molecules. That the receptors were intact and functional was shown by the fact that they responded normally to GABA and to the benzodiazepines when these substances were applied to the surface of the oocytes. This remarkable demonstration raises considerably the reliability of the proof

that the correct stretches of DNA had indeed been cloned.

The second step was to show that there are strong homologies (similarities in DNA sequence) between the receptor for GABA and the receptor for acetylcholine, which is an important excitatory transmitter. The conclusion drawn by Barnard and his colleagues is that both receptors belong to a "superfamily" of receptor molecules, which is very old in evolutionary terms. One intriguing implication of this hypothesis is that the receptors for both excitatory and inhibitory transmitters may well be descended from a common molecular ancestor.

Thinking about the evolutionary descent of inhibitory neurotransmitters naturally raises the question of their function. Clearly, inhibitory activity, which is so widespread in the brain and spinal cord, must fulfill a significant function. It has long been thought that the inhibitory neurons act collectively as a governor that prevents excitatory neurons from firing to excess. There is some evidence that the inhibitory nerve cells do indeed carry out this function. For example, the administration to experimental animals of agents that block the effect of GABA (such as picrotoxin or bicuculline) triggers widespread excess neural activity accompanied by convulsions.

Yet this rather passive, nonspecific activity is certainly not the whole story, as some interesting recent work has shown. Since picrotoxin and bicuculline selectively block GABAergic synapses, it is possible to apply these compounds and examine how neural networks operate with their GABAergic synapses silenced. My colleagues John H. Caldwell, Harry J. Wyatt and Nigel W. Daw took that approach with the rabbit retina. It had already been shown by Horace B. Barlow of the University of California at Berkeley that many of the ganglion cells in the rabbit retina—which are the cells that relay visual information to the brain—are directionally selective: they respond to a stimulus moving, say, from left to right but not to one moving from right to left.

Daw and his co-workers examined the responses of such ganglion cells before, during and after the application of picrotoxin. They found that in the presence of picrotoxin the directional sensitivity was erased—the ganglion cells responded equally well to a stimulus moving in either direction—only to reappear when the drug was washed out of the tissue.

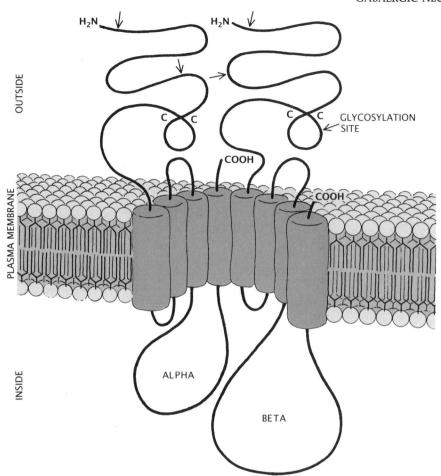

Figure 75 GABA RECEPTOR twines through the outer membrane of the postsynaptic cell. The receptor consists of two subunits, designated alpha and beta. Each subunit is a long chain of amino acids that includes four helical regions, which probably form a channel for chloride ions. Arrows indicate points where sugar molecules are attached to the amino acid chain. This model was proposed in 1987 by E. A. Barnard of the U.K. Medical Research Council's Molecular Neurobiology Unit and co-workers.

The most plausible explanation of these remarkable results is that a GABAergic neuron endows the ganglion cell with its directional sensitivity. Light striking the retina activates photoreceptors (called rods and cones) that trigger the ganglion cells only through the intermediate effects of cells called bipolar cells. Branches of the bipolar cells also excite GABAergic neurons called amacrine cells, whose processes are arranged horizontally and make contact with the ganglion cells. A certain subset of amacrine cells must be arranged asymmetrically, so that when they are stimulated, they inhibit ganglion cells to the left or the right, but not both (see Figure 76). In the presence of picrotoxin, the amacrine cell's effect

is blocked, and the ganglion cell responds to movement in either direction.

Thus the amacrine cell gives the rabbit's retina a key feature: the capacity to detect the direction of movement. It is not difficult to see how such sensitivity could be of great evolutionary benefit in judging the motions of predators or other objects. Similar benefits may come from another effect of the GABAergic neurons, which has been examined by Robert W. Dykes of McGill University and his colleagues, who worked with cats.

Healthy cats are capable of distinguishing very well between stimuli quite close together on their skin. They are able to do so because certain neurons

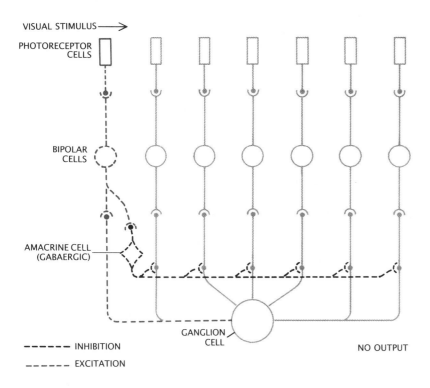

VISUAL STIMULUS ⟶

PHOTORECEPTOR CELLS

BIPOLAR CELLS

AMACRINE CELL (GABAERGIC)

GANGLION CELL

NO OUTPUT

- - - - - - INHIBITION

- - - - - - EXCITATION

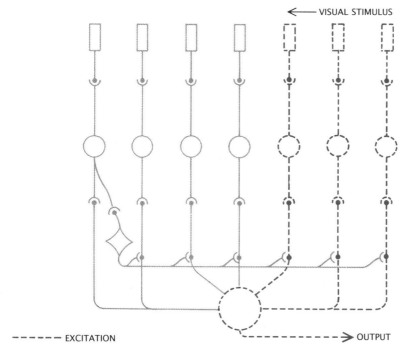

⟵ VISUAL STIMULUS

- - - - - EXCITATION

⟶ OUTPUT

Figure 76 NETWORK OF PHOTORECEPTOR CELLS in the retina responds to changes in light intensity and passes its signal to bipolar cells, whose responses converge onto ganglion cells. If a stimulus moves from left to right (*top*), the first photoreceptor cell excites a bipolar cell (*broken line*), which triggers a GABAergic amacrine cell. The GABAergic neuron silences the other bipolar cells and the ganglion cell is silent. The bipolar cells on the other side of this network, however, are not wired to the amacrine cell (*bottom*). A stimulus that is moving from right to left activates the ganglion cells.

in the brain respond to stimuli only within a highly circumscribed area, which is called their receptive field. These neurons are concentrated within a structure called the somatosensory cortex. When bicuculline is injected into the somatosensory cortex, the receptive fields of many of the neurons expand dramatically beyond their normal limits. As in the case of the rabbit retina, the effect is reversible, disappearing after the drug is removed.

The best explanation for these effects is, again, that GABAergic neurons are selectively canceling sensory inputs. It would seem that neurons in the somatosensory cortex actually receive excitatory inputs from a large area on the skin surface. Not all the inputs from that area, however, are created equal. Those from the peripheral region are accompanied by inhibitory inputs that cancel their effects, whereas those from the central region pass through uninhibited, thereby defining the small region of sensitivity.

These two examples show clearly that the role of inhibitory neurons in general, and GABAergic neurons in particular, goes far beyond regulating overall levels of activity in the manner of a neuronal governor. In their newly understood capacity as specifiers of responsiveness they may be of fundamental significance to the operation of the brain. Modern concepts of brain function stress that intricate neural networks are the basis of the brain's capacity to sift and analyze the information supplied by the senses. By tuning the responsiveness of key neurons, the GABAergic neurons may shape the networks, and so, as much as the excitatory pathways, form the basis of sentience and action.

Neuropeptides

They are short chains of amino acids that are active in the nervous system. In some cases they transmit signals between nerve cells and also serve the body as a hormone.

· · ·

Floyd E. Bloom

October, 1981

The two major systems that coordinate the activity of cells with the needs of the body have long been thought to function in quite different ways. In the nervous system each nerve cell has been taken to affect its set of target cells at synapses: specialized sites at which a chemical messenger—a neurotransmitter—is released by one cell and received by another. In many instances the neurotransmitter is a monoamine: a substance the nerve cell synthesizes by making minor changes in an amino acid. Sometimes the neurotransmitter is the amino acid itself. In any case its release and reception take milliseconds. In short, such communication is point-to-point and fast. In the endocrine system, on the other hand, each gland cell has long been known to release its chemical product—a hormone—into the circulating blood. The hormone is often a peptide: a short chain of amino acids. The release of the hormone, its circulation in the blood and its influence on its target cells throughout the body takes minutes or hours.

These distinctions between the two systems are now in disarray. For one thing norepinephrine, a monoamine neurotransmitter, turns out to be also a hormone: it is released by gland cells in the medulla of the adrenal gland. Conversely, vasopressin, a peptide hormone, turns out to be also a neurotransmitter: nerve cells in the hypothalamus, a part of the brain, rely on vasopressin to signal other nerve cells in the brain. Today more than a dozen cell-to-cell messengers are known to be capable of relaying signals either between nerve cells or between gland cells and their targets. Typically each messenger is discovered first as a factor: a substance of unknown chemical composition that has a physiological effect such as the dilation of arteries or the contraction of muscle. Often it emerges that the factor is made up of amino acids. Then it emerges that the factor is active in the brain. Thus the factor is revealed as a neuropeptide.

The discovery of a peptide messenger begins with the suspicion that a chemical substance is responsible for the interaction of two groups of cells. For example, it has long been known that if an animal is anesthetized with ether, the cortex of the adrenal gland releases steroid hormones in quantity. If the anterior lobe of the pituitary gland is first removed, no such release is measured. Presumably, therefore, a substance released by the anterior lobe causes the adrenal cortex to act. The substance turns out to be adrenocorticotrophic hormone, or ACTH, also called corticotropin. In a different experiment the blood vessels linking the hypothalamus to the anterior lobe of the pituitary are interrupted. Again the etherization of the animal does not give rise to the release of steroids. Evidently the hypothalamus governs the release of pituitary corticotropin. The substance by which it does so is called corticotropin releasing factor. Its molecular structure has not yet been worked out.

THE PROCESS OF DISCOVERY

The suspicion that two groups of cells interact by means of a chemical messenger motivates a sequence of experiments that is well established today. The sequence was devised largely by Vincent du Vigneaud of the Cornell University Medical College as he worked in the 1940's and 1950's to identify the hormones secreted by the posterior lobe of the pituitary. It was elaborated in the 1960's and 1970's by Roger Guillemin, who is now at the Salk Institute for Biological Studies, and by Andrew V. Schally, who is now at the New Orleans Veterans Administration Hospital. The objects of their search were the hormones by which the hypothalamus regulates the anterior lobe of the pituitary.

First an extract is prepared from the group of cells that presumably release a factor. This can be done, for example, by homogenizing the cells. The extract is applied to the tissue whose cells the factor controls. The potency of the extract is noted; then the extract can be refined by passing it through a chemical sieve consisting of a gel that selectively filters molecules on the basis of their size or their electric charge. The refined extract is applied to the tissue. With skill, and often with luck, one finds that it now has greater potency than the original extract had. The factor has therefore been concentrated. Further refinements of the extract are tested for potency. Ultimately the factor is purified. In some instances the process begins with extracts from hundreds of thousands of fragments of brain and ends with a few nanograms of an unknown chemical substance.

At this point a different technology is applied to the factor to determine its chemical structure. Suppose the factor is inferred to be a peptide because it loses its biological activity when it is treated with enzymes that cleave peptide chains at the linkages between two successive amino acids. A chemical assay then shows the proportions of the various amino acids. The precise sequence of amino acids remains to be determined. The classical technique is to treat the factor with a number of enzymes each of which cleaves the peptide chain at the linkages between two specific amino acids.

The resulting fragments are collected. Individual amino acids are successively cleaved from each one and identified by properties such as the rate at which they travel in a column of gel that filters molecules according to their electric charge. In this way the sequence of amino acids in each fragment is worked out. Next the order of the fragments themselves is determined by finding overlapping sequences of amino acids in the sets of fragments cleaved from the factor by enzymes that cleave a peptide at different sites. The newest technique removes amino acids from the full peptide chain one by one; a mass spectrometer then identifies each amino acid in the sequence by its weight.

When a sequence has been determined, its proportional content of the various amino acids is matched against the composition of the factor as it has been determined by chemical assay. Then the peptide is synthesized. Today this can be done readily; indeed, a peptide is often commercially available within weeks of its discovery. The quantity of the synthetic replicate is much greater than the quantity investigators could hope to produce by progressive purifications of a cell extract. Hence the replicate can be tested to see if it matches the purified natural peptide in both action and potency. Moreover, the replicate can be tested for biological activity on tissues other than the one it is known to act on.

Further still, the replicate can be injected into an animal of a species other than the one from which the peptide was purified. The immune system of the animal will prime antibodies against the peptide. The peptide itself can be quite short; thus its sequence of amino acids may be nearly identical in many species. In such instances the priming of antibodies is encouraged by linking the peptide to a large carrier molecule before it is injected. In any case the antibodies have several uses. In the technique called the radio-immunoassay, developed by Solomon A. Berson and Rosalyn S. Yalow of the Bronx Veterans Administration Hospital, they are mixed with a replicate of the peptide in which some of the atoms are radioactive. The antibodies bind to the replicate. Then a tissue extract is added to the mixture. The native peptide in the extract will displace a certain amount of the replicate. The degree of displaced radioactivity is a sensitive measure of the amount of native peptide.

The antibodies can also serve as a microscopic stain to reveal the location of cells that store the peptide and presumably utilize it. In some techniques the antibody is labeled with a chemical group that is fluorescent or one that is radioactive. In still other techniques the antibody is linked to an enzyme that can manufacture a pigment inside cells. The most elaborate staining technique calls for animals of three different species. Suppose a peptide has been purified from the brain of a rat and a synthetic replicate of the peptide has been prepared. The replicate is injected into a rabbit. The resulting rabbit antibodies are applied to sections of the brain of a rat. There they bind to the native peptide. The rabbit antibodies are also injected into a goat. The result is goat antibodies that act against rabbit antibodies. These goat molecules are labeled and applied to the sectioned rat brain. They bind to the rabbit antibody, which is already bound to the peptide. The double-antibody technique has the advantage that the antibody prepared against the synthetic peptide is not subjected to a chemical labeling reaction, which might alter its ability to react with the native peptide molecule.

The employment of antibodies to seek out the peptide often reveals that many more cells contain the peptide than had been thought. Indeed, certain peptides have been found in neurons that were known to contain a monoamine and so had been taken to be specialized for the release of that neurotransmitter alone. At the same time the elucidation of the chemical structure of the factor often makes possible an improvement in the method used to purify the natural factor from the cells that contain it. If the factor is a peptide, for example, and the original method of purification began with a homogenate of brain tissue, it may well be that the disruption of the cells by the homogenization allowed the peptide to be attacked by the enzymes called peptidases. A method can then be devised in which such enzymes are inactivated before the peptide is extracted. Sometimes the result is surprising: a larger form of the peptide is discovered. It had gone undetected because the first extraction procedure had destroyed it. In some instances the larger peptide is more potent than the smaller one.

VASOPRESSIN AND OXYTOCIN

As more and more peptides have been purified and their structure has been determined several groups of chemically related substances have emerged. Two types of group can be distinguished. In one type the peptides purified from cells across a wide range of species include almost identical long sequences of amino acids. In the second type a number of different large peptides purified from the cells of a single species include identical short sequences of amino acids. Presumably the sequences that are identical have proved particularly well suited for intercellular signaling through long periods of evolution.

Consider the peptide messengers first identified by du Vigneaud and his colleagues as factors released by the posterior lobe of the pituitary gland, an appendage to the brain. They can be seen in the gland as fatty droplets inside the terminals of the axons, or long fibers, of nerve cells in the hypothalamus. To Ernst A. Scharrer, who was then at the University of Colorado School of Medicine, the cells seemed to be typical neurons: they appeared to get information from their synapses with other cells. Scharrer thus advanced the surprising hypothesis that the cells were neurosecretory neurons: like any other nerve cell they were controlled by synaptic connections, and yet on suitable command they could secrete a hormone into the bloodstream. It is now recognized that their axons also project to several levels of the brain. Hence they evidently rely on the hormone as a neurotransmitter. Working at the Albert Einstein College of Medicine in New York, Berta V. Scharrer, Ernst's widow, found similar neurons in the nervous system of a number of invertebrate species.

Du Vigneaud named the factors in accord with their physiological action. Specifically, he distinguished a factor he called antidiuretic hormone, which acts on the kidneys of an animal deprived of drinking water to lessen the loss of water in the urine, and a factor called oxytocin, which promotes the contraction of the muscle of the uterus and thereby speeds birth. When it emerged that antidiuretic hormone could elevate the blood pressure by causing certain arteries to constrict it, the factor was given the second name vasopressin.

Vasopressin and oxytocin turn out, then, to be an example of a family of peptides whose structure is well conserved across a wide range of species. In most vertebrate animals less advanced than the

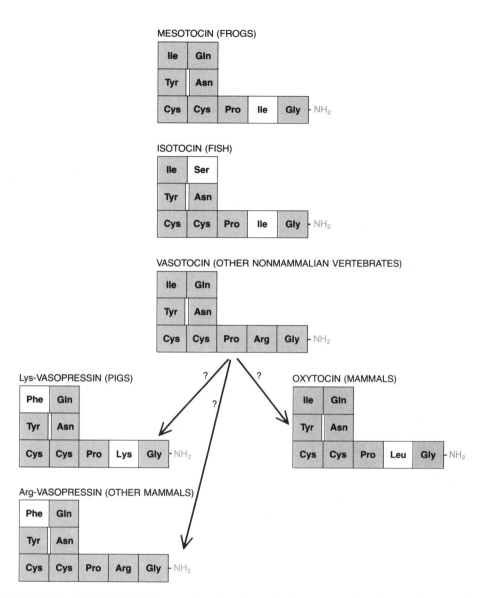

Figure 77 VASOPRESSIN AND OXYTOCIN are released by the nerve cells in the hypothalamus of mammals from the posterior lobe of the pituitary gland. Both are almost identical in structure with vasotocin, mesotocin or isotocin (top), the hormones released from the posterior lobe in nonmammalian vertebrate animals. The similarities (color) suggest that vasopressin and oxytocin arose through mutations in duplicate copies of a single gene.

mammals the family is represented by a single substance, which is called arginine-vasotocin because of the presence of the amino acid arginine at position No. 8 in its chain of amino acids. In mammals the hormones oxytocin and vasopressin appear. Oxytocin is identical with vasotocin except that the amino acid leucine takes the place of arginine at position No. 8. Vasopressin is slightly more idiosyn-

cratic. In all mammals except the pig it is identical with vasotocin except that phenylalanine substitutes for isoleucine at position No. 3. In the pig one finds two substitutions: lysine takes the place of arginine at position No. 8 and phenylalanine takes the place of isoleucine at position No. 3.

Wilbur H. Sawyer of the Columbia University College of Physicians and Surgeons has conjectured that a gene duplication may have allowed a peptide modified at position No. 8 to evolve from arginine-vasotocin. The modification would lessen the peptide's antidiuretic action and enhance its oxytocic action. In any case the alteration in the action of a peptide hormone because of a minor change in the structure of the peptide shows that each peptide acts on different target cells in spite of the small degree of difference. It follows that the receptors on the target cells (that is, the sites on the membrane of the target cells that "recognize" the messenger) must be precise enough to accept the one molecule and reject the other. Perhaps some further minor modifications of the molecules will yield synthetic peptides whose specificity of action is greatly enhanced. Such substances might well be valuable pharmaceuticals.

ENDORPHINS AND ENKEPHALINS

Perhaps the most striking example of the second type of family relationship among peptide messengers—the presence of certain short sequences of amino acids common to several coexistent peptides—is provided by the endorphins and the enkephalins. The terms have emerged from a decade of almost frenzied research; they are now taken to signify classes of brain peptides whose effects on cells resemble those of opiates such as morphine. (The word endorphin is a contraction of endogenous morphine.) The saga of the endorphins and the enkephalins began with the discovery in several laboratories, including those of Solomon H. Snyder at the Johns Hopkins University Medical School, Eric J. Simon at the New York University School of Medicine and Lars Terenius at the University of Uppsala, that certain cells in the brain have receptors that bind opiates. Some of the cells lie in brain structures implicated in the perception of pain; others, however, do not. Then Hans W. Kosterlitz and John R. Hughes of the University of Aberdeen purified from brain-cell extracts a fraction that occurs naturally in the brain and suppresses the contraction of muscle tissue from the intestine, much like morphine itself. The molecules with this action turned out to be two pentapeptides. One of them has the sequence tyrosine-glycine-glycine-phenylalanine-methionine; it is known as met-enkephalin. The other, which is identical except that leucine substitutes for methionine, is leu-enkephalin.

Soon the met-enkephalin sequence was found in a number of longer peptides purified from an endocrine gland: the anterior lobe of the pituitary. Then the longer peptides—the endorphins—were found

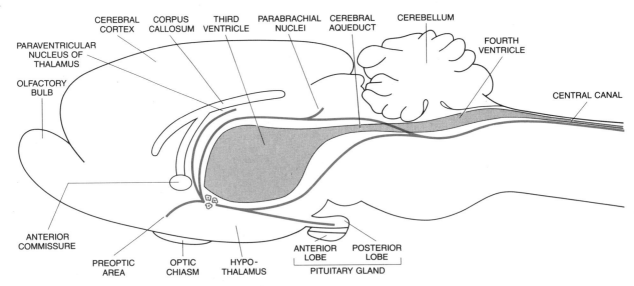

Figure 78 NERVE CELLS EMPLOYING OXYTOCIN as their neurotransmitter are found in the rat's supraoptic nucleus and paraventricular nucleus of the hypothalamus. The axons of the cells project into the posterior lobe of the pituitary gland, from which they release the oxytocin as a hormone. They also project into cell groups in the brain and spinal cord.

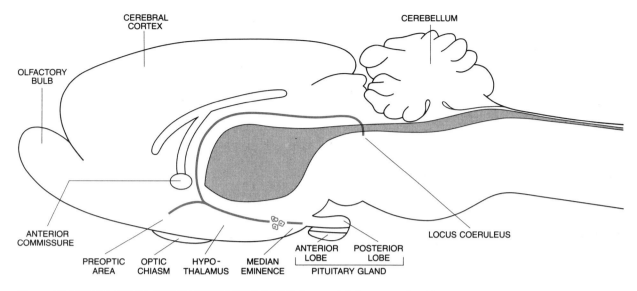

Figure 79 NERVE CELLS CONTAINING ENDORPHIN are found in the rat in the arcuate nucleus of the hypothalamus. The axons of the cells (see also Figure 78) project along pathways in the brain similar to those of the cells containing oxytocin. The pattern shown emerges also for corticotropin and gamma-MSH, two other peptide messengers in the precursor pro-opiomelanocortin.

also in nerve cells. Some investigators surmised that such nerve cells shorten an endorphin to make an enkephalin. The hypothesis was contradicted, however, by the preparation of antibodies to the endorphins and the enkephalins and the subsequent mapping of the nerve cells that contain them. The staining patterns reported for the enkephalins by Tomas G. M. Hökfelt and his associates at the Karolinska Institute in Sweden show that cells containing enkephalins are widespread in the brain. They lie, for example, in the spinal cord, the brain stem, the hippocampus and the corpus striatum. In con-

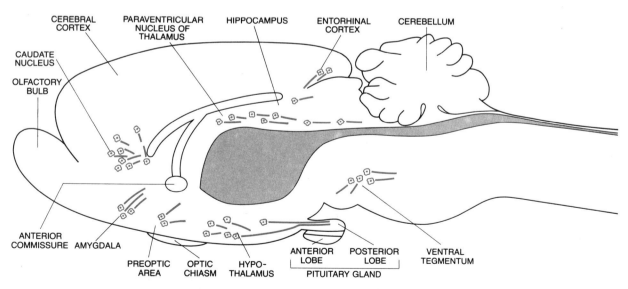

Figure 80 NERVE CELLS CONTAINING ENKEPHALIN are widespread in the brain of the rat, which makes them distinct from the nerve cells containing endorphin. Here the cells containing enkephalin are projected onto the midplane of the brain and displayed in proportion to the actual numbers of such cells at various locations. The trajectories of the axons arising from the cells are suggested by line segments.

trast the staining patterns my colleagues and I at the Salk Institute have found for the endorphins place them exclusively in nerve cells at the base of the hypothalamus and in endocrine cells in the anterior lobe of the pituitary.

The family relations being discovered within the endorphins and within the enkephalins are becoming complex and distinctive. For the endorphins the first hint of complexity came when Richard Mains and Betty Eipper of the University of Colorado and Nicholas Ling of the Salk Institute discovered why endorphins are found in the cells of the anterior pituitary that release the hormone corticotropin. Each such cell makes a long precursor peptide from which a molecule of endorphin and a molecule of corticotropin are cleaved. The precursor was given the provisional name pro-opiocortin. Yet it was twice as long as it would be if it consisted of a molecule of corticotropin joined to a molecule of endorphin.

Quite recently the entire sequence of amino acids that make up the precursor has been determined by Stanley N. Cohen of the Stanford University School of Medicine and Shosaku Numa and Shigetada Nakanishi of the Kyoto University Faculty of Medicine. These workers determined the sequence without attempting to purify the peptide as in the orthodox process of discovery. Instead they employed the new techniques of genetic engineering to produce multiple copies of the messenger RNA that specifies the sequence. Then they worked out the structure of the messenger RNA. The RNA is a strand of the units called nucleotides. A particular triplet of nucleotides encodes the identity of a particular amino acid.

In the wake of the work of this group it proved advisable to call the precursor pro-opiomelanocortin. The added term melano refers to a sequence of seven amino acids. One copy of the sequence is included in corticotropin; it is called alpha-melanocyte stimulating hormone (alpha-MSH) because it is known to disperse the pigment melanin in the pigment cells (melanocytes) in the skin of the frog. It thereby modulates the color of the skin. (When a green frog is placed in the dark, its skin turns brown.) A nearly identical sequence lies next to the endorphin sequence in pro-opiomelanocortin; it is called beta-MSH. It was discovered by Choh Hao Li of the University of California at San Francisco, who purified a number of pituitary peptides and determined their sequences of amino acids by classical methods in the late 1950's and early 1960's.

What Cohen, Numa and Nakanishi discovered was a third sequence almost identical with the other two. It lies in the section of the pro-opiomelanocortin chain whose sequence of amino acids had not previously been determined. The third sequence was named gamma-MSH in advance of any evidence that it has its own action in the body. Work done at the Salk Institute by Ling and Guillemin and their colleagues and by my colleagues and me suggests, however, that gamma-MSH is stored in cells of the anterior lobe of the pituitary. Moreover, when gamma-MSH is injected into a cerebral ventricle of an experimental animal (a fluid-filled space in the brain), the animal's body temperature decreases. Evidence is also accumulating that certain cells of the hypothalamus rely on gamma-MSH as a neurotransmitter.

MOLECULES INCORPORATING ENKEPHALIN

The complexities in the enkephalin branch of the family are also increasing now that investigators in the U.S. and Japan have begun to detect enkephalin sequences in longer molecules that are otherwise unlike the endorphins. The differences lie in the amino acids next to the end of the enkephalin pentapeptide designated the C terminus. Specifically, the endorphins in pro-opiomelanocortin have serine and threonine in that position, whereas the recently discovered molecules that incorporate the enkephalin sequence have lysine and arginine there. Lysine and arginine are special amino acids in that they each have two amino (NH_2) groups, one of which projects from the amino acid's molecular structure. Studies of a large number of peptides show that the sites where two such amino acids are adjacent in the peptide chain are the places where enzymes most often cleave the peptide. The two adjacent amino

Figure 81 PEPTIDE MESSENGERS (in amino acid sequence in cattle). The pro-opiomelanocortin chain incorporates the chains of corticotropin (1-39) and beta-lipotropin (42-132). The corticotropin chain incorporates the chains of alpha-MSH (1-13) and of CLIP, or corticotropin-like intermediate-lobe peptide (18-39). Beta-lipotropin incorporates gamma lipotropin (42-99), beta-MSH (82-99) and beta-endorphin (102-132). Five amino acids at one end of the endorphin chain (102-106) duplicate the sequence of an enkephalin. Ends of gamma-MSH may lie at a bond between the amino acids arginine and lysine (−57 and −56) and a bond between two arginines (−43 and −42), places where enzymes that cleave peptide chains typically act.

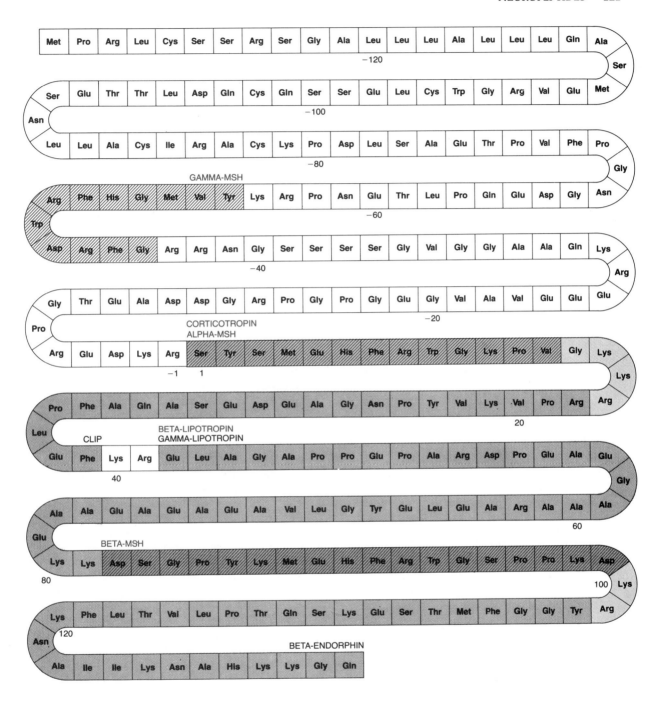

Met	Pro	Arg	Leu	Cys	Ser	Ser	Arg	Ser	Gly	Ala	Leu	Leu	Leu	Ala	Leu	Leu	Leu	Gln	Ala

−120

Ser · Ser | Glu | Thr | Thr | Leu | Asp | Gln | Cys | Gln | Ser | Ser | Glu | Leu | Cys | Trp | Gly | Arg | Val | Glu | Met

−100

Asn · Leu | Leu | Ala | Cys | Ile | Arg | Ala | Cys | Lys | Pro | Asp | Leu | Ser | Ala | Glu | Thr | Pro | Val | Phe | Pro

−80

GAMMA-MSH

Gly · Arg | Phe | His | Gly | Met | Val | Tyr | Lys | Arg | Pro | Asn | Glu | Thr | Leu | Pro | Gln | Glu | Asp | Gly | Asn

−60

Trp · Asp | Arg | Phe | Gly | Arg | Arg | Asn | Gly | Ser | Ser | Ser | Ser | Gly | Val | Gly | Gly | Ala | Ala | Gln | Lys

−40

Arg · Gly | Thr | Glu | Ala | Asp | Asp | Gly | Arg | Pro | Gly | Pro | Gly | Glu | Gly | Val | Ala | Val | Glu | Glu | Glu

−20

CORTICOTROPIN
ALPHA-MSH

Pro · Arg | Glu | Asp | Lys | Arg | Ser | Tyr | Ser | Met | Glu | His | Phe | Arg | Trp | Gly | Lys | Pro | Val | Gly | Lys

−1   1

Lys · Pro | Phe | Ala | Gln | Ala | Ser | Glu | Asp | Glu | Ala | Gly | Asn | Pro | Tyr | Val | Lys | Val | Pro | Arg | Arg

20

CLIP   BETA-LIPOTROPIN
GAMMA-LIPOTROPIN

Leu · Glu | Phe | Lys | Arg | Glu | Leu | Ala | Gly | Ala | Pro | Pro | Glu | Pro | Ala | Arg | Asp | Pro | Glu | Ala | Glu

40

Glu · Ala | Ala | Glu | Ala | Glu | Ala | Glu | Ala | Val | Leu | Gly | Tyr | Glu | Leu | Glu | Ala | Arg | Ala | Ala | Ala

60

BETA-MSH

Glu · Lys | Lys | Asp | Ser | Gly | Pro | Tyr | Lys | Met | Glu | His | Phe | Arg | Trp | Gly | Ser | Pro | Pro | Lys | Asp

80 ... 100

Asn · Lys | Phe | Leu | Thr | Val | Leu | Pro | Thr | Gln | Ser | Lys | Glu | Ser | Thr | Met | Phe | Gly | Gly | Tyr | Arg

120

BETA-ENDORPHIN

Ala | Ile | Ile | Lys | Asn | Ala | His | Lys | Lys | Gly | Gln

Ala Alanine	**Gly** Glycine
Arg Arginine	**His** Histidine
Asn Asparagine	**Ile** Isoleucine
Asp Aspartate	**Leu** Leucine
Cys Cysteine	**Lys** Lysine
Gln Glutamine	**Met** Methionine
Glu Glutamate	**Phe** Phenylalanine

Pro Proline	
Ser Serine	
Thr Threonine	
Trp Tryptophan	
Tyr Tyrosine	
Val Valine	

groups protruding from the peptide chain may well be the feature the enzyme recognizes when it binds to the peptide and cleaves it. The occurrence of the feature next to the enkephalin pentapeptide suggests that the large molecules are precursors of enkephalin.

One version of a large molecule that includes leu-enkephalin was discovered recently by Avram S. Goldstein and his colleagues at the Stanford School of medicine. They call it dynorphin because it is more potent than enkephalin in the standard biological assay for the effect of an opiate. (In the standard assay the substance is applied to a sample of smooth muscle from the intestine of a guinea pig. The muscle is induced to contract by electrical stimulation, and the degree of the substance's ability to suppress the contraction constitutes the assay.) Other large molecules that include enkephalins are also reported to be more potent than the enkephalin sequence itself. Thus it is conceivable that the first estimates of the potency of the enkephalins were based on studies of the partially degraded larger forms.

Still another complication in the enkephalins arose when Hökfelt and his colleagues applied the immunohistochemical stains for the enkephalins to the cells of the adrenal medulla. The cells were previously known to secrete only the monoamines epinephrine and norepinephrine. Now Hökfelt's group found that these cells show a large degree of what Hökfelt was careful to call "enkephalin-like" reactivity to the stain. He was cautious in his conclusions because he considered it possible that the antibody employed for the staining procedure had bound itself not to enkephalin but to a similar sequence in some undiscovered peptide.

The caution was well placed. A series of discoveries made in laboratories including that of Sidney Udenfriend at the Roche Institute of Molecular Biology has now revealed that several large peptides from extracts of the adrenal medulla include the enkephalin sequence. One of them is at least 10 times larger than enkephalin. It has several copies of the met-enkephalin sequence and at least one copy of leu-enkephalin. The large polyenkephalin peptides seem to be secreted in tandem with epinephrine and norepinephrine but at less than a hundredth the concentration. Moreover, no interaction between the peptide messengers and the monoamine messengers on a common target cell has yet been discovered.

GUT PEPTIDES IN THE BRAIN

The nerve cells that include the pro-opiomelanocortin peptide present a special problem: Do they pare that precursor down into an endorphin, into corticotropin or into gamma-MSH, or do they pare it down into other peptide molecules not yet known to be messengers? Perhaps the signals arriving at such a cell can direct the cleaving of the precursor so that certain axon terminals release specific products.

A related problem then arises. The enkephalins and some of the endorphins suppress the perception of pain. Hence it has sometimes been advanced that the modulation of the perception of pain is their primary function. The enkephalins and the endorphins are now found, however, in brain circuits that are implicated in a wide range of functions, including the control of blood pressure and body temperature, the regulation of the secretion of hormones and the governance of body movement. This wide range of functions has confounded the effort to attribute to the messengers a single domain of function.

To be sure, it might be advanced that several independent systems depend on messengers that share the amino acid sequence of an enkephalin. Presumably the messengers share the sequence because they evolved from some single messenger early in animal evolution. Today each such system would act on a different set of target cells; thus each set of target cells would require its own type of receptor, and a given type of receptor would have to be able to distinguish between two molecules that differ only slightly in structure.

The view that the various systems exploiting enkephalins and endorphins might be independent was presaged by William D. Martin of the University of Kentucky Medical Center well before the endorphins were discovered. His study of the actions of opiates on the spinal cord of the dog had shown that different actions of morphine are simulated or blocked by different drugs. This suggested distinct classes of opiate receptors. More recently the work of Kosterlitz at Aberdeen, Albert Herz at the Max Planck Institute for Psychiatry in Munich, Goldstein at Stanford and several other investigators shows that the various peptides containing an enkephalin pentapeptide differ considerably in their potency in suppressing the perception of pain or the contractility of smooth muscle. This too suggests several classes of receptors.

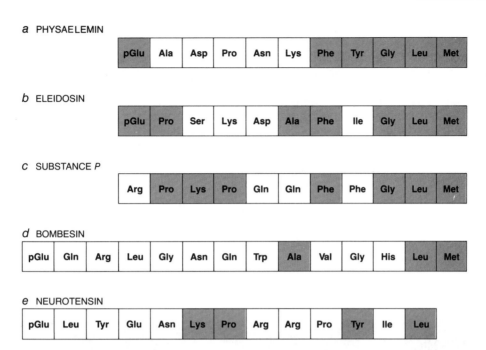

a PHYSAELEMIN

| pGlu | Ala | Asp | Pro | Asn | Lys | Phe | Tyr | Gly | Leu | Met |

b ELEIDOSIN

| pGlu | Pro | Ser | Lys | Asp | Ala | Phe | Ile | Gly | Leu | Met |

c SUBSTANCE *P*

| Arg | Pro | Lys | Pro | Gln | Gln | Phe | Phe | Gly | Leu | Met |

d BOMBESIN

| pGlu | Gln | Arg | Leu | Gly | Asn | Gln | Trp | Ala | Val | Gly | His | Leu | Met |

e NEUROTENSIN

| pGlu | Leu | Tyr | Glu | Asn | Lys | Pro | Arg | Arg | Pro | Tyr | Ile | Leu |

Figure 82 PEPTIDES RESEMBLING PHYSAELEMIN form a family of perhaps as many as five. Physaelemin (*a*) has been purified from frog skin, eleidosin (*b*) from the salivary glands of the octopus. Substance *P* (*c*), bombesin (*d*) and neurotensin (*e*) have been purified from the nervous system of mammals. All five substances promote the contraction of muscle tissue from the viscera, but it is not known if they act that way in the body. Color denotes duplications of amino acids and pGlu stands for pyroglutamate, which appears at the same end of four of the peptides.

Adopting (at least for the moment) the view that the cells secreting structurally similar peptides need not be functionally related may help to explain why many peptides once thought to serve only the gut or the endocrine system are also detected in the brain. Often they are found in parts of the brain that have nothing to do with the realm in which the substance acts in the periphery of the body. Among these substances are the peptides of the gut (and now the brain) called substance *P*, vasoactive intestinal peptide and cholecystokinin. Each one has been found in neurons that make local synaptic connections ("local-circuit neurons") in the cerebral cortex and in the hippocampus. Moreover, nerve fibers containing substance *P* or vasoactive intestinal peptide have been found innervating visceral tissues such as parts of the lung. They have even been found innervating the thyroid gland, where no nerve fibers were known to terminate.

A still more striking example of an almost ubiquitous peptide messenger is somatostatin. It is a substance that Paul Brazeau, Wyley Vale, Roger C. Burgus and Ling and Guillemin of the Salk Institute discovered by applying the classical process of discovery to extracts from the hypothalamus. The biological assay they resorted to as a criterion for successive purification of the extract was the ability of each successive extract to suppress the secretion of growth hormone by cells these workers had cultured from the anterior lobe of the pituitary. Soon it was determined that somatostatin is a peptide consisting of 14 amino acids. Then a replicate of somatostatin was synthesized and antibodies to it were developed. The employment of the antibodies as a stain placed somatostatin in certain cells of the hypothalamus positioned so that they can secrete the substance into a system of capillaries that carries it into the anterior lobe.

Further studies of the distribution of somatostatin have been little less than astounding. In the nervous system somatostatin is found in nerve cells in almost every neural tissue from the cerebral cortex to the autonomic ganglia: the nests of nerve cells in the periphery that govern the tissues of the viscera. In the gut somatostatin is found in the cells that line the intestine. In the endocrine system somatostatin is found in the delta cells of the islets of Langerhans. Its action in the pancreas appears to suppress the secretion of the hormones insulin and glucagon. Quite recently larger forms of somatostatin have been extracted from the pancreas and the brain that are more potent than the sequence of 14 amino acids.

PEPTIDES AS NEUROTRANSMITTERS

The utilization of a peptide by a nerve cell as a neurotransmitter differs from the utilization of an amino acid or a monoamine in a fundamental respect: the way the nerve cell synthesizes the substance and conserves it. A neurotransmitter such as gamma-aminobutyrate, serotonin or dopamine is made in a short series of steps from an amino acid in the diet. For each step an enzyme in the cytoplasm of the cell acts as a catalyst. In general each nerve cell includes the enzymes that synthesize a single transmitter. The active form of the transmitter molecule is stored in the sacs called synaptic vesicles until the nerve cell is called on to release it. After the transmitter is released the cell can reabsorb some of it. In that way the need for the synthesis of the transmitter is somewhat reduced.

In a cell that releases a peptide the process is more involved. In the first place the peptide can be synthesized only by ribosomes, the specialized intracel-

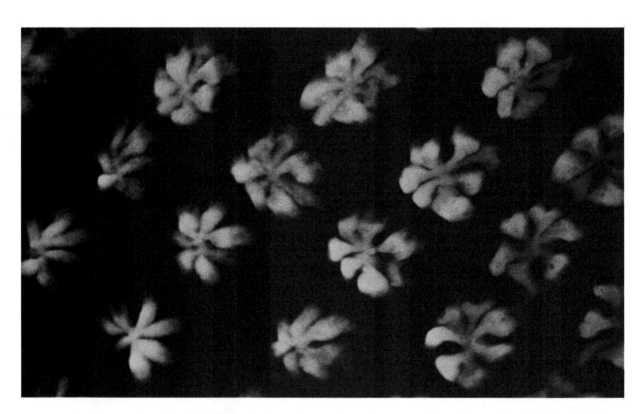

Figure 83 PRESENCE OF ENKEPHALIN in the organ of sight of several species is demonstrated by a technique that tags the enkephalin with an antibody and then tags the antibody with a second antibody to which a fluorescent molecule is bound. The enkephalin itself is a neuropeptide consisting of five amino acids. The photo shows a retinula, or sight organ, of the lobster. The fluorescence marks sprays of cells. Each spray is an ommatidium, a cluster of light receptors some 10 micrometers in diameter. (Photo by J. Mancillas and J. F. McGinty of the Salk Institute.)

lular organelles that synthesize all peptides, including the long ones: proteins. This means the sequence of amino acids that make up the peptide must be encoded by a gene, a strand of DNA in the nucleus of the cell. The gene must be transcribed into a strand of messenger RNA, which carries the code to the ribosome. In the second place all the peptide neurotransmitters examined so far appear to follow the pattern of the endorphins in that it seems they are synthesized first as a larger peptide. Then the active form of the molecule is produced through progressive cleavages by enzymes.

The ribosomes in a nerve cell lie only in the cell body and in the filamentous extensions of the cell body called dendrites. In general, however, the dendrites and the cell body of a nerve cell receive signals from other cells. A longer filament, the axon, transmits signals to other cells. Hence the release of a peptide neurotransmitter from an axon terminal is remote from the place where the peptide is made. The active form of the peptide (stored in synaptic vesicles) must be transported, then, to the place of release. It may follow that a cell releasing a peptide is unable to act on another cell repeatedly in a short span of time. In contrast, the axon terminals of a cell that releases an amino acid or a monoamine may well be satellite factories that make their own transmitter. Such terminals may stand less in need of replenished supplies of fresh neurotransmitter from moment to moment.

A further way in which a peptide neurotransmitter may differ from a monoamine neurotransmitter lies in the molecular details of how the transmitter influences its target cells. The classical neurotrans-

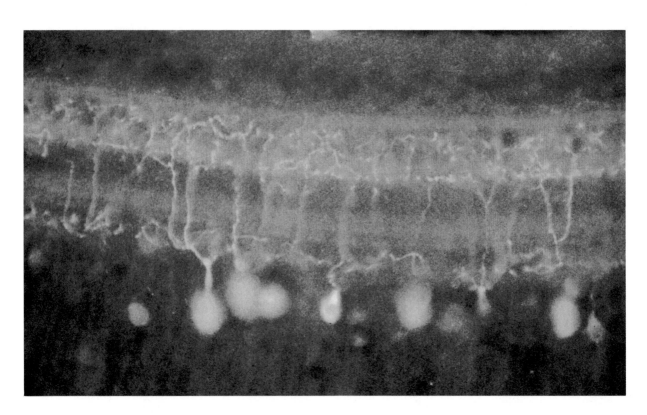

Figure 84 CELLS CONTAINING ENKEPHALIN in the retina of a chick are nerve cells, not light receptors. Each cell belongs to the class of neurons called amacrine cells, which make local connections in the retina by means of filaments that the demonstration technique renders fluorescent. Some of the amacrine cells not marked by fluorescence in this preparation turn out to contain other neuropeptides: neurotensin, substance *P*, somatostatin or vasoactive intestinal peptide. (Photo by N. Brecha and H. J. Karten at the State University of New York at Stony Brook.)

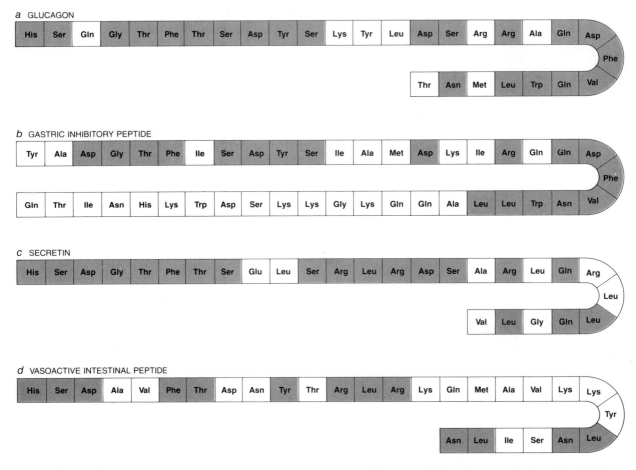

a GLUCAGON

| His | Ser | Gln | Gly | Thr | Phe | Thr | Ser | Asp | Tyr | Ser | Lys | Tyr | Leu | Asp | Ser | Arg | Arg | Ala | Gln | Asp |

Phe

| Thr | Asn | Met | Leu | Trp | Gln | Val |

b GASTRIC INHIBITORY PEPTIDE

| Tyr | Ala | Asp | Gly | Thr | Phe | Ile | Ser | Asp | Tyr | Ser | Ile | Ala | Met | Asp | Lys | Ile | Arg | Gln | Gln | Asp |

Phe

| Gln | Thr | Ile | Asn | His | Lys | Trp | Asp | Ser | Lys | Lys | Gly | Lys | Gln | Gln | Ala | Leu | Leu | Trp | Asn | Val |

c SECRETIN

| His | Ser | Asp | Gly | Thr | Phe | Thr | Ser | Glu | Leu | Ser | Arg | Leu | Arg | Asp | Ser | Ala | Arg | Leu | Gln | Arg |

Leu

| Val | Leu | Gly | Gln | Leu |

d VASOACTIVE INTESTINAL PEPTIDE

| His | Ser | Asp | Ala | Val | Phe | Thr | Asp | Asn | Tyr | Thr | Arg | Leu | Arg | Lys | Gln | Met | Ala | Val | Lys | Lys |

Tyr

| Asn | Leu | Ile | Ser | Asn | Leu |

Figure 85 PEPTIDES RESEMBLING GLUCAGON form a family of four. Glucagon (*a*) is a hormone synthesized by the alpha cells of the islets of the pancreas. Gastric inhibitory peptide (*b*) has been purified from the lining of the stomach. Secretin (*c*) has been purified from the lining of the small intestine. Vasoactive intestinal peptide (*d*), first purified from the lining of the small intestine, has turned up in nerve fibers that innervate the intestine and in the brain. Duplications of amino acids in the family are shown in color.

mitters are said to be excitatory or inhibitory. The arrival of molecules of an excitatory neurotransmitter makes the target cell more likely to release its own neurotransmitter from its own axon terminals; the arrival of an inhibitory neurotransmitter has the opposite effect. Investigators who have studied these actions emphasize that the neurotransmitter alters the permeability of the target cell's membrane to ions of potassium, sodium or calcium. As a result of such changes the concentration of these ions inside the target cell changes with respect to their concentration outside the cell. The differing concentrations give rise to a voltage gradient across the membrane. The action of an excitatory neurotrans-

mitter tends to diminish the voltage gradient; it "depolarizes" the membrane. The action of an inhibitory transmitter tends to increase the voltage gradient; it "hyperpolarizes" the membrane.

In experiments with the enkephalins, substance *P* and other peptide messengers a different action appears. The peptide makes the target cell less likely to respond to other signals. One might consider this to be an example of inhibition. In some instances, however, the peptide messenger keeps an excitatory transmitter from depolarizing the membrane; in other instances it keeps an inhibitory transmitter from hyperpolarizing it. Moreover, the arrival of the peptide itself often produces no notable change in

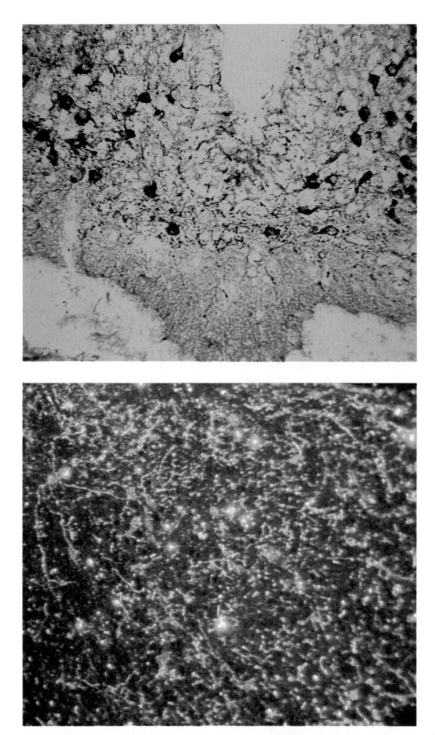

Figure 86 PRESENCE OF BETA-ENDORPHIN, a neuro-peptide, is demonstrated in the arcuate nucleus in the rat hypothalamus by a technique that employs antibodies to tag the cells containing beta-endorphin. The upper photo shows the preparation under the light microscope. The brown pigment marks numerous nerve cells. They appear to be the only cells in the brain of the rat that contain beta-endorphin. The lower photo shows the tissue under dark-field illumination. The varicosities that show up in gold are axons and dendrites. The cell bodies themselves are small, elongated triangles. Bluish pinpoints of light are irregularities at the tissue's surface. (Photos by E. Batten-berg and the author at the Salk Institute.)

the voltage gradient across the membrane. This curious effect of a peptide messenger is one I like to call disenabling. It has now been reported by Roger Nicoll of the University of California at San Francisco, who studied peptides in the spinal cord of the frog; by Jeffrey L. Barker and his colleagues at the National Institute of Neurological and Communicative Disorders and Stroke, who studied enkephalin in the mammalian neurons they cultured from the spinal cord; by Walter Zieglgänsberger and his colleagues at the Max Planck Institute for Psychiatry, who studied enkephalin in the spinal cord of the cat, and by Zieglgänsberger and George R. Siggins at the Salk Institute, who studied enkephalin in slices of hippocampus of the rat.

Since the peptide and the disenabled transmitter must each act on the target cell at a different set of receptors, one imagines the two sets of receptors might interact. Indeed, it seems that certain small populations of nerve cells can release both a monoamine and a peptide. Some are thought to release both acetylcholine and vasoactive intestinal peptide, others to release both dopamine and cholecystokinin and still others to release both serotonin and substance *P*. The arrival of such a pair of messengers at a target cell might give rise to a complex sequence of effects.

THE MEDIATION OF BEHAVIOR

The ultimate question about any intercellular messenger is how it integrates the activities of cells in a way that is appropriate to the circumstances in which the organism finds itself. Briefly, how does it mediate behavior? One answer is suggested by the work of Donald Pfaff and his colleagues at Rockefeller University and that of Robert L. Moss and Samuel M. McCann at the Southwestern Medical School of the University of Texas Health Science Center in Dallas. In each case the work concerns the decapeptide called luteinizing hormone releasing hormone (LHRH). LHRH is a substance purified from the hypothalamus that causes the release of luteinizing hormone from the anterior lobe of the pituitary. Luteinizing hormone in turn induces ovulation. LHRH has now been found in nerve cells in the autonomic ganglion that innervates the reproductive organs. Its utilization there instead of some other messenger may be fortuitous. As it happens, however, the injection of LHRH into a male or female rat either subcutaneously or into a cerebral ventricle evokes the posture required for copulation. It is as if several activities that constitute reproductive behavior were coordinated by the same peptide messenger.

A further example of the mediation of behavior by a peptide is the ability of angiotensin II to bring on drinking behavior. The work of James T. Fitzsimons and his colleagues at the University of Cambridge shows that the injection of a few nanograms of angiotensin II under the skin or the injection of a few picograms into a cerebral ventricle causes behavior indistinguishable from spontaneous drinking in species ranging from lizards to primates. The animal's water balance or salt balance seems not to matter.

The discovery of angiotensin's behavioral effect adds to a considerable list of its physiological effects. Basically the events that activate angiotensin begin when any of three circumstances (low blood pressure, a low local concentration of sodium or direct stimulation by nerve fibers) causes certain cells in the kidney to secrete the enzyme renin. In the bloodstream renin acts on a protein manufactured in the liver and liberates a decapeptide called angiotensin I. In the bloodstream or in any of several organs including the brain a second enzyme cleaves two amino acids off from angiotensin I. An octapeptide remains. It is angiotensin II. Its physiological effects include the constriction of blood vessels supplying the skin and the kidneys, the dilation of blood vessels supplying muscles and the brain and an increase in blood pressure.

In addition angiotensin II causes the adrenal cortex to increase its output of aldosterone, a hormone that acts in turn on the kidneys to cause the reabsorption of sodium from the urine. Further still, angiotensin II increases the secretion of vasopressin from the posterior lobe of the pituitary. Vasopressin then promotes the reabsorption of water from the urine. All these actions tend to reverse the trends that triggered the secretion of renin. Thus they regulate three aspects of the blood: its volume, its pressure and its content of sodium. The fact that angiotensin II elicits drinking behavior is consistent with all its other effects.

According to the findings of Ian R. Phillips, who is now at the University of Florida, the cells in the brain that detect angiotensin are curious neurons in the hypothalamus and the brain stem that line the ventricles. Each one sends an extension of its cell body into a ventricle and yet each maintains typical synaptic connections with other neurons. The neurons they contact presumably include the neurons in the hypothalamus that secrete vasopressin. Remarkably, the subcutaneous or intraventricular injection of vasopressin does not elicit drinking behavior even when the experimental animal is dehydrated and presumably thirsty. On the other hand, the effects of circulating angiotensin do not account for every episode of drinking behavior. If they did, the behavior and the blood level of angiotensin would be linked. The work of Edward M. Stricker of the University of Pittsburgh suggests that this correlation is sometimes lacking. Doubtless the motivation to drink and the motor acts involved in seeking water and drinking it call for the simultaneous activity of several linked brain systems.

Although vasopressin does not cause animals to drink, it is reported to have effects on behavior that are even more dramatic. Over the past decade David de Wied and his colleagues at the State University of Utrecht and Abba J. Kastin and his colleagues at the New Orleans Veterans Administration Hospital have reported observations that vasopressin and other peptides affect learning and memory. In one experimental arrangement rats were taught not to enter a dark box by being given an electric shock whenever they did. They were reported to continue to avoid the box for a longer period after the end of the training if they were given a subcutaneous injection of a minute amount of vasopressin. Molecular segments of corticotropin or of endorphin that have no known neural or endocrine actions were said to have the same property.

A TEST OF VASOPRESSIN

Together with Michel Le Moal of the University of Bordeaux, George F. Koob and I set out three years ago to test the effects of vasopressin and other peptides on behavior. We resorted to an arrangement of de Wied's in which rats were trained to jump onto a pole whenever a light bulb lit up in warning that a painful electric shock was about to be delivered through the floor. When the training was complete, the light would be lit from time to time but no shock would be delivered. Before the training began we gave one group of rats an intraventricular injection of a saline solution; in general they stopped jumping onto the pole within four hours after the end of

the training. We injected a second group of rats with a solution containing a nanogram of vasopressin; they continued to jump for eight to 10 hours after the end of the training. Strangely, a third group of rats, each given 50 nanograms of vasopressin, stopped jumping before the control group. It was as if the extra vasopressin had helped them to see through our ruse.

The change in behavior brought on by vasopressin seems, then, to be unquestionable. It is not clear, however, that the change represents the action of vasopressin on the unknown cellular processes that underlie learning and memory. The change may have a simpler explanation. In view of the effects of vasopressin on the circulatory system we were not surprised to find that even low doses of vasopressin caused brief but immediate elevations of blood pressure. We were sent a synthetic analogue of vasopressin by Sawyer of the Columbia College of Physicians and Surgeons and Maurice Manning of the Medical College of Ohio in Cincinnati. The analogue prevents vasopressin from elevating blood pressure. The rats to which the analogue was administered along with vasopressin showed no change in blood pressure, and they behaved like the control group.

The altered performance of the rats under the influence of vasopressin could mean, therefore, that the rats were aroused by an unnatural and unnecessary elevation of blood pressure and remained tense and alert for hours. The rats were aroused, that is, by a change in the body that the brain did not request. This seems less impressive than the hypothesis that vasopressin mediates learning and memory directly. On the other hand, a mismatch between the brain's commands and the body's responses may be sufficient to invoke behavioral strategies for dealing with novel situations. People given long-lasting analogues of vasopressin report enhanced attention to their surroundings, and their performance on tests of memory improves.

Moreover, even on the simpler hypothesis a neuropeptide apparently serves to signal that the survival of the animal is challenged and that the animal had best be attentive to its surroundings. Conversely, the absence of such a signal may suggest that the animal is momentarily safe. Survival signals such as these could represent a means by which the neuropeptides guide the evolution of complex forms of behavior. Surely the various aspects of research on peptide messengers are likely to advance understanding both of cellular regulation and of the means by which certain types of animal behavior result from decipherable cell-to-cell interactions.

POSTSCRIPT

Since 1981 more peptides have been sequenced and their metabolic pathways studied (Lynch and Snyder, 1986). In fact, the entire armamentarium of molecular biology has been brought to bear on these rather small molecules, and their study has advanced our understanding of the means by which diversity is generated during evolution (Schwartz and Costa, 1986). However, the picture of their localization is not totally clear (Chan et al., 1984). The location of gut-brain peptides is controversial; those native to one site may not necessarily be found in the other. It is also not known what determines where a peptide will be expressed or which will have endrocrine and which a neurotransmitter function. Investigations using new techniques such as cDNA probes are progressing to determine where the various peptides are synthesized, but these techniques will not reveal the meaning of peptide localization. The action of peptides has also received much attention and this picture is becoming quite complex. A peptide may have many independent actions, which may be quite different from those with which it was originally associated (Kastin and Zadina, 1986).

The Functional Architecture of the Retina

Dozens of kinds of cells have specialized roles in encoding the visual world. New techniques have made it possible to study the arrangement and interconnections of entire populations of cells.

. . .

Richard H. Masland

December, 1986

The retina encodes the visual world. It transforms optical images into trains of nerve impulses, which are then conducted along the optic nerve to the brain. The brain interprets those signals to generate visual perception: a subjective sense of the shapes, colors and movements that surround the observer. The retina is more than just a bank of photocells, however. This thin sheet of neural tissue at the back of the eye is an outpost of the central nervous system. Its circuits of interconnected neurons, or nerve cells, carry out a form of image analysis: certain features of the raw visual input are accentuated and other features are downplayed.

The effort to understand how light signals are transduced into neural activity and how that activity is transformed has intrigued neurobiologists for many years. The general nature of the retina's encoding of the visual world—the relation of its output to its input—was established first. A skeletal view of the means by which the coding is accomplished was attained by the early 1970's. The retina was known to be composed of five main classes of neurons. They are connected to one another by synapses: points of close apposition where the chemical messengers called neurotransmitters are released by one neuron to affect the next neuron. Three of the five classes of retinal neurons form a direct pathway from the retina to the brain. These are the photoreceptors (the rod cells and cone cells), the bipolar cells and the ganglion cells. The remaining two classes of retinal neurons, the horizontal and the amacrine cells, form laterally directed pathways that modify and control the message being passed along the direct pathway.

Until recently it seemed that these five classes of cells exactly defined the retina's functional elements. Each class of cells was thought to carry out a single kind of task; to understand the retina's internal codes, neurobiologists should have only to decipher the interactions of these relatively few basic elements. Now, instead, it has become clear that the retina has many more than five functional elements. The five cell classes harbor subtypes so distinctive that the true number of functional elements may be as high as 50.

The task, then, is to learn why so many cell types are required. It is very far from having been com-

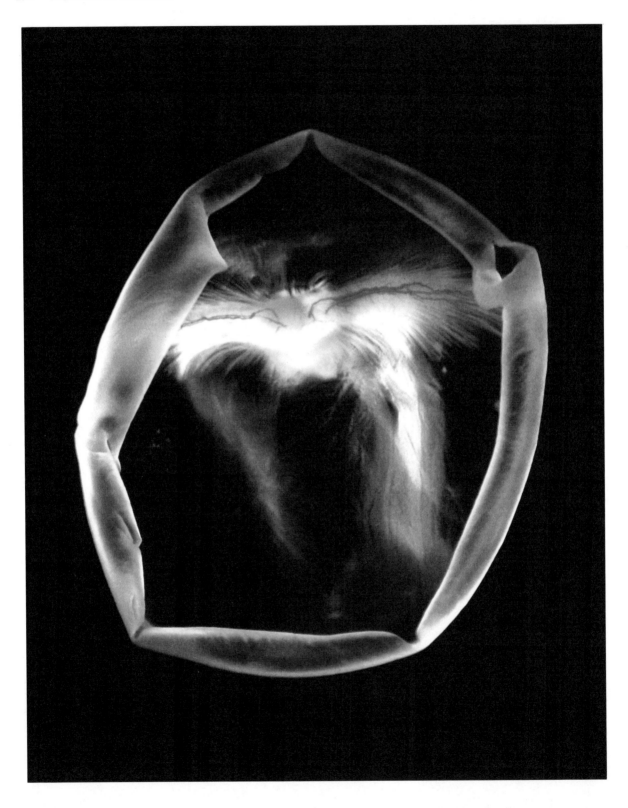

Figure 87 ISOLATED RABBIT RETINA, a sheet of neural tissue lining the inside of the back of the eye whose average thickness is only about a tenth of a millimeter, is essentially transparent. Light passes through it to strike the rod and cone cells near its back surface. These photoreceptors transduce the light signal into a neural signal, which is relayed by successive layers of retinal neurons; ultimately the signal excites ganglion cells, whose axons form fibers (*white filaments*) that join to form the optic nerve. Two pairs of blood vessels are seen crossing the front surface of the retina. Methods for isolating the living retina from the eye were first developed by Adelbert Ames III. (Photograph by the author.)

pleted, but in the past few years important progress has been made. A significant advance has been the development of ways to examine the shapes and the arrangement in the retina of entire populations of nerve cells.

An understanding of precisely how the mammalian retina codes visual information began in 1952 with a series of experiments on ganglion cells,

the cells whose axons form the optic nerve. These first experiments, carried out by Stephen W. Kuffler at the Johns Hopkins University School of Medicine, sought to answer the question: How does the electrical activity of ganglion cells change in response to light? Kuffler recorded the electrical activity of single ganglion cells. He found that most of them fire a continuous stream of action potentials, or nerve impulses, along their axons even in the absence of light. A ganglion cell responds to the presence of light by markedly increasing or decreasing its rate of firing.

Mapping the surface of the retina of anesthetized cats with small spots of light, Kuffler stimulated specific regions of the retina and measured the electrical response of individual cells. He found that each ganglion cell has a precise area of the visual field to which it responds: its receptive field. The size of the receptive field varies, but it is generally quite small. In the cat the centers of the smallest receptive fields occupy a region of the retina about 120 micrometers (thousandths of a millimeter) in

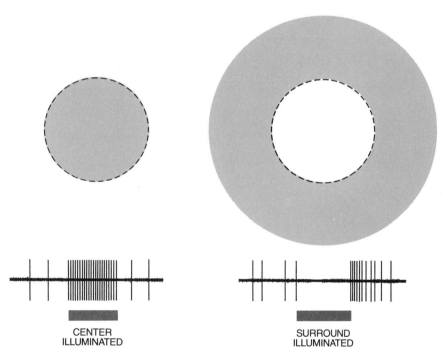

CENTER
ILLUMINATED

SURROUND
ILLUMINATED

Figure 88 CONCENTRIC RECEPTIVE FIELD has a central region in which stimulation by light has one effect on a ganglion cell's firing (recorded by a microelectrode measuring the activity of a single axon in the optic nerve) and a surrounding region in which the effect is the opposite (*top*). In the case of an on-center cell, stimulation of the center causes an increase in activity (*bottom left*), stimulation of the surround a decrease (*bottom right*).

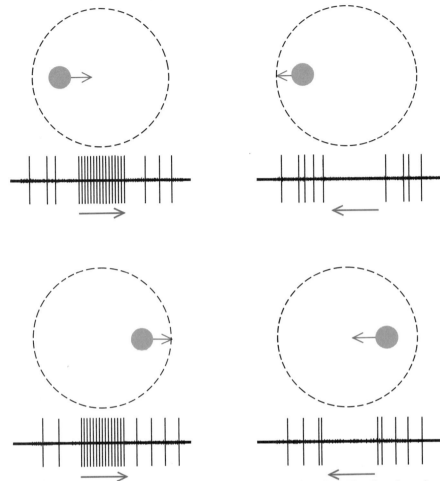

Figure 89 DIRECTIONALLY SELECTIVE CELL responds when a spot moves in one direction (to the right in the diagram) and is inhibited when the spot moves in the opposite direction. The direction of movement is detected wherever the spot may fall in the receptive field.

diameter. If the cat looks at a wall two meters away, each such ganglion cell reports on an area roughly a centimeter in diameter.

The cells Kuffler studied can be divided into two populations: those that are stimulated and those that are inhibited when the center of their receptive field is stimulated. Moreover, the centers act in opposition to the region encircling them: the surround. If stimulation of the receptive field's center excites the cell, stimulation of the surround inhibits it. Conversely, if the center is inhibited by light, the surround is excited by it. In other words, the surround is "antagonistic"; the cell carries out a simple form of contrast enhancement.

A very different kind of ganglion cell was soon identified: the directionally selective cell, whose receptive field responds to the direction of a moving stimulus. (It turned out to be only one of a series of cells having complex stimulus selectivities, but it is the most abundant and well studied of them and can serve as a prototype.) Directionally selective cells were discovered in the frog by Jerome Y. Lettvin, Humberto R. Maturana, Walter H. Pitts and Warren S. McCulloch of the Massachusetts Institute of Technology. It was not until several years later, however, that the exact properties of these cells were elucidated in a series of classical experiments carried out on rabbits by Horace B. Barlow and

William R. Levick of the University of Cambridge.

The behavior of a directionally selective cell varies depending on whether the light stimulus is moving or stationary. If one maps the cell's receptive field with a stationary light, the cell responds uniformly throughout its receptive field. When a spot of light is moved slowly across the cell's receptive field, however, the behavior of the cell changes dramatically: it fires a sustained train of action potentials when the spot moves in one direction and fires little or not at all when the spot moves in the opposite direction. These early results defined basic questions about retinal circuits. What establishes a ganglion cell's receptive field? How can neuronal machinery transform the optical input so selectively? To find answers one must look at the retina's internal components in more detail.

A s I mentioned above, the retina can be said to have two sets of neurons: those that establish a direct pathway from the source of light to the optic nerve and those that make lateral connections. It was immediately obvious that the antagonistic surround observed for some ganglion cells could be accounted for if the retina's laterally conducting neurons function in opposition to the through-pathway neurons. In other words, when the center of a ganglion cell responds to light (by way of the direct pathway), its surround (which acts in opposition) might be driven by stimuli transmitted by way of horizontal or amacrine cells. A role for horizontal cells received crucial support when it was learned that bipolar cells have antagonistic surrounds. Since the bipolar cell is the only cell that conducts from the outer retina (where horizontal cells reside) to the

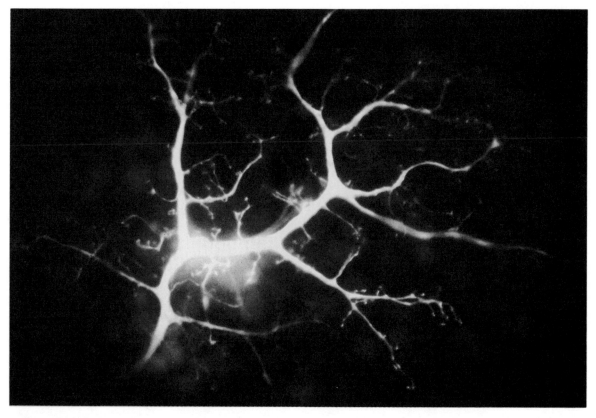

Figure 90 RETINAL NEURON, a horizontal cell, was injected with the fluorescent dye Lucifer Yellow, which stains all the cell's processes. A terminal arborization of the cell is seen in the micrograph. Information flows later- **ally along such a cell's branches and small twigs to the buttonlike terminal boutons, which make synaptic contact with other cells in the retina. (Micrograph by J. H. Sandell.)**

inner retina, no other machinery was needed to explain the existence of antagonistic surrounds.

Other lateral neurons, the amacrine cells, regulate the behavior of certain ganglion cells (including the directionally selective ones) that exhibit a transient response to stimulation by light. When light strikes the retina, these cells immediately fire a burst of action potentials, but they cease firing in the presence of continued light stimulation. Transient behavior is not exhibited to this degree by photoreceptor, bipolar or horizontal cells. It is, however, characteristic of many of the amacrine cells. One role of amacrine cells, then, is presumably to sharpen the transient responses of certain ganglion cells, including the directionally selective ones.

Amacrine cells must have more roles than that, however. These cells come in a bewildering variety; a single retina may contain as many as 30 morphologically distinct types. If amacrine cells had no function other than to make the response of some ganglion cells transient, one might reasonably expect there to be only one kind of amacrine cell, or certainly no more than a few kinds.

The diversity of amacrine cell shapes had been reported as far back as 1892 by the great Spanish neuroanatomist Santiago Ramón y Cajal. For a long time his findings were disregarded. Among other possibilities, one could always argue that the different cell shapes he described were merely variants: cells that look different but have the same function. It was not until the late 1960's, when Berndt Ehinger of the University of Lund in Sweden began studying amacrine cell biochemistry, that the true

diversity of amacrine cells was recognized. Ehinger applied to the retina newly developed methods for identifying neurotransmitters in thin sections of neural tissue. He found that a large number of the neurotransmitters known to be present in the brain were also present in retinal neurons. The surprising thing was that all these neurotransmitters were found in one or another amacrine cell, each neurotransmitter in a subset of the amacrine cells. This implied that there are many distinct subsets of amacrine cells.

At first Ehinger's results were viewed with some skepticism. The methods were new, and one could argue that they had overestimated or underestimated the amacrine cell populations. Yet subsequent studies by other investigators led to the same results. Among these was a study, carried out by John W. Mills and me at Massachusetts General Hospital, of amacrine cells that synthesize the neurotransmitter acetylcholine. We incubated isolated rabbit retinas in the presence of radioactively labeled choline, the precursor from which the cells synthesize acetylcholine. Our next objective was to immobilize acetylcholine for autoradiography (a method for localizing radioactivity in tissue sections) so that we could determine which cells had synthesized acetylcholine. To do this we used a fast-freezing method. Samples of living retinas were plunged directly into propane at −180 degrees Celsius, the tissues were freeze-dried and then prepared for autoradiography by methods that keep them from coming into contact with moisture.

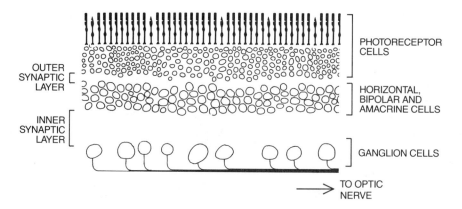

Figure 91 RETINAL-NEURON CELL BODIES are arranged in three layers. In addition there are two synaptic layers, where the processes of the cells (axons and dendrites) intertwine and make synaptic contact with one another.

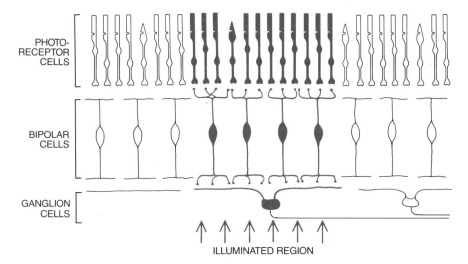

Figure 92 RETINA'S PRIMARY THROUGH PATHWAY is provided by three kinds of neurons: photoreceptor cells, bipolar cells and ganglion cells. A retina composed of these cells could transmit information about light, but its ganglion cells would display no selective features; they would have only a "center" response.

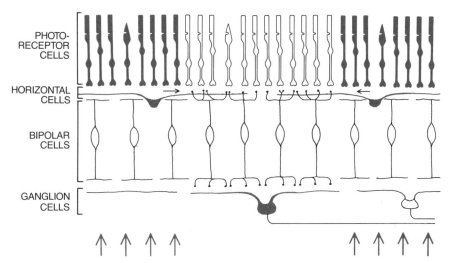

Figure 93 LATERAL INTERACTIONS can account for such selective features as a receptive field's antagonistic surround. Suppose the horizontal cells have an effect (*black arrows*) on the bipolar cells that is opposite to the direct effect of the photoreceptor cells. Then the final sig- nals transmitted to a ganglion cell will have a center and an antagonistic surround. The actual horizontal-cell connections that mediate this effect are still incompletely known.

These methods are tedious, but they have a special advantage: the tissue's acetylcholine is immobilized within a few milliseconds by the freezing. When it is subsequently located by autoradiography, it must still be within the cell where it originally belonged. The technique thus eliminates some

of the uncertainties that attended earlier methods for identifying neurotransmitters in cells. The labeling was sharp and distinctive: a cell was either densely labeled or not labeled at all. Acetylcholine was present only in a very small subset of amacrine cells. As time went on, other laboratories also confirmed Ehinger's fundamental finding. As he had suggested, different neurotransmitters are confined to small subsets of amacrine cells.

Knowing this, one could try to link particular neurotransmitters to morphologically distinct types of amacrine cells, such as those described by Ramón y Cajal. It was quickly learned that amacrine cells having differently shaped dendritic trees could be matched with particular neurotransmitters. Among the evidence, moreover, was work by Nicholas C. Brecha and Harvey J. Karten of the State University of New York at Stony Brook showing that not only the traditional neurotransmitters but also many of the body's neural peptides (a large family of newly discovered peptide neurotransmitters) are present in distinct amacrine cells. This finding increased the diversity of amacrine cells beyond all expectations.

The discovery that shape and synaptic chemistry are interrelated in amacrine cells had a second and crucially important consequence. It removed any remaining doubt that amacrine cells having different shapes have different biological functions. When a neurotransmitter binds to a receptor on a postsynaptic cell, that cell undergoes specific biochemical and physiological changes. If various amacrine cells have both different shapes (which imply different connections within the retina) and different neurotransmitters, they must have differing biological roles. What role could 30 different amacrine cells possibly have? Each type undoubtedly has its specific function, but there seem to be far more kinds of cells than there are jobs for them to do. In my laboratory and in others some of these jobs are now beginning to be revealed. Here I shall describe work with four very different amacrine cells.

The first of these cells has already been mentioned. It is the cholinergic, or acetylcholine-containing, amacrine cell that was identified by autoradiography. One drawback to autoradiography was that it reveals the cell body of a neuron but not

the processes: the axons and dendrites that transmit and receive messages. In fact, the major anatomical method for seeing the processes was the Golgi technique—the very method Ramón y Cajal used in the 19th century. That method cannot be controlled: it stains an entire cell, but the investigator cannot choose the cell ahead of time.

A substitute for the Golgi technique was suggested by my discovery that a fluorescent molecule, 4,6-diamidino-2-phenylindole (DAPI) accumulates selectively in the cell bodies of the cholinergic neurons. If one treats an entire retina with DAPI and then mounts the retina flat, the cholinergic neurons fluoresce beautifully against the darker background. This made it possible for Masaki Tauchi, a postdoctoral student, and me to guide a fine micropipette to a cell and inject it with a different fluorescent dye, Lucifer Yellow CH. The Lucifer Yellow diffuses through the cell's entire network of branches. The results were perfectly consistent: all the fluorescent cells had the same shape and branching pattern.

This method not only showed us the true shape of the cholinergic cells but also enabled us to reconstruct the mosaic they form as they blanket the retina. To see why this was important one must again think about the job the retina does. The retina must, above all, preserve spatial resolution; any failure would compromise the acuity with which the animal can see. The density and spatial arrangement of the retina's intermediate elements—through which visual information must pass—thus provide important information about the role those elements can play within the system as a whole. Pioneering analyses of retinal cell mosaics had been done by Brian B. Boycott and Heinz Wässle at King's College London for two cells that can be stained as entire populations by classical methods. Our fluorescence methods make it possible to study many other cells.

When Tauchi and I measured the size and density of the cholinergic cells, we found a surprising result.

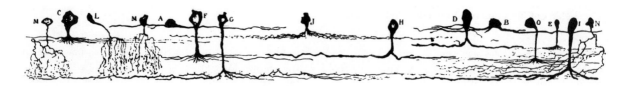

Figure 94 WIDE VARIETY of amacrine cells is displayed in this drawing, published in 1892 by the Spanish neuroanatomist Santiago Ramón y Cajal, of amacrine cells in the carp retina. He was able to distinguish 14 cell types on the basis of their shape alone.

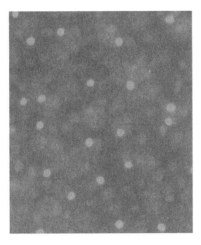

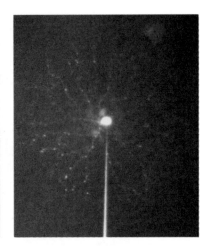

Figure 95 CHOLINERGIC AMACRINE CELLS. A retina is mounted flat as an intact sheet. The cholinergic amacrine cell bodies selectively accumulate DAPI, a blue fluorescent dye (left). This makes it possible to guide a micropipette that has been filled with another dye, Lucifer Yellow CH, into an individual amacrine cell under illumination that makes both dyes fluoresce (center). Under different illumination (right) only the Lucifer Yellow fluoresces, revealing the distinctive branching pattern of the cholinergic cell's dendrites.

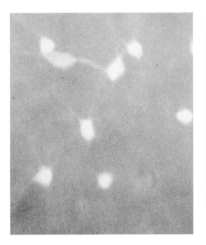
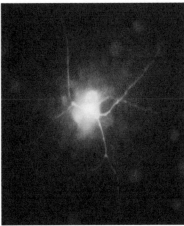
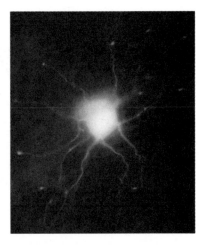

Figure 96 TWO OTHER AMACRINE CELL TYPES are stained by the same method described in Figure 95. A retina was treated in such a way that the cell bodies of dopaminergic amacrine cells fluoresce in green, those of indoleamine-accumulating amacrine cells in yellow (left). Injection of individual cells shows the specific dendritic shapes of dopaminergic cells (center) and indoleamine-accumulating cells (right).

The cells overlap one another a great deal. In the peripheral retina, where the overlap is greatest, a point on the retinal surface is overlaid by the processes of some 140 cholinergic amacrine cells. Boycott and Wässle's work had suggested that the overlap would be slight. Such enormous redundancy was entirely unexpected.

A possible explanation for the redundancy was suggested by the kinds of stimuli the cholinergic amacrine cells can resolve. From previous electrophysiological work we knew that cholinergic amacrine cells excite certain ganglion cells, among them the directionally selective ones. We knew that these ganglion cells can detect the movement of very small spots—spots smaller than their dendritic field. The spots are also much smaller than the dendritic field of the cholinergic amacrine cells. Because most neurons simultaneously transmit the same message across all their synapses, an amacrine cell would be expected to release acetylcholine from all points on its dendritic tree whenever any one point was excited. How can a cell that is so spread out transmit precise information about stimuli smaller than itself?

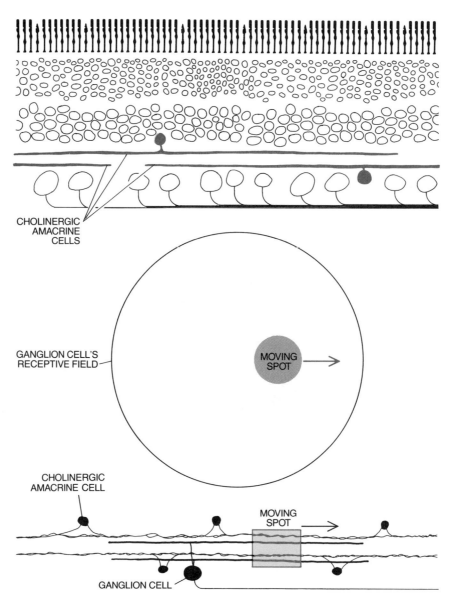

CHOLINERGIC
AMACRINE
CELLS

GANGLION CELL'S
RECEPTIVE FIELD

MOVING
SPOT

CHOLINERGIC
AMACRINE CELL

MOVING
SPOT

GANGLION CELL

Figure 97 RESOLUTION of the cholinergic amacrine cell may be explained by the fact that its dendrites are both input and output processes and can act in isolation from the rest of the cell. Cholinergic amacrine cells are shown schematically (*color*) in a vertical section of the full retina (*top*). The edges of a moving spot in a ganglion cell's receptive field (*middle*) excite only particular regions of the mosaic of amacrine cell dendrites (*bottom*); the cholinergic dendrites thereupon excite the ganglion cell only in the illuminated region.

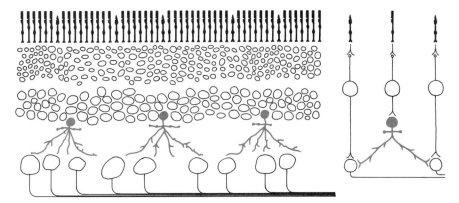

Figure 98 AII AMACRINE CELL (*color*) is positioned between rod-driven bipolar cells and ganglion cells (*left*). It provides a bridge between a rod-driven bipolar cell and a ganglion cell (*right*). The cell's connections are shown schematically; an AII amacrine cell actually is connected to different types of ganglion cell by different pathways.

Our best guess is that the dendrites of the amacrine cell are electrically isolated, enabling one region to release acetylcholine to a ganglion cell locally without there being any release at more distant sites. This is consistent with the structure of amacrine cells, in which inputs and outputs exist side by side on the same process. The electrical activity of the cholinergic amacrine cells consists only of graded electric potentials; the cells do not generate nerve impulses, which would propagate throughout their dendritic trees. The activity should therefore not spread much beyond the point of input. Although direct proof that this mechanism exists is currently beyond our capabilities, there seems to be no other way to explain the resolution of the directionally selective cell. Moreover, such a mechanism makes the tight meshwork of cholinergic amacrine cell dendrites an actual advantage: a small stimulus can be detected no matter where it may fall within the ganglion cell's receptive field.

The second type of amacrine cell I shall describe is the AII cell, which differs from the cholinergic cell in that it has an extremely narrow lateral spread. David Vaney of the University of Cambridge was able to describe the mosaic formed by AII cells by adapting our fluorescence-guided injection method. These cells are abundant and cover the entire surface of the retina, but they are so small that their dendrites do not overlap much.

Several other workers have studied AII cells, including Helga Kolb and Ralph F. Nelson of the National Institutes of Health, Barbara A. McGuire,

Peter Sterling and John K. Stevens of the University of Pennsylvania School of Medicine and Ramon F. Dacheux and Elio Raviola of the Harvard Medical School. As a result of their painstaking work there is now an answer to a question posed several years ago by Kolb and Edward V. Famiglietti: How can ganglion cells fire in response to dim light even though they do not receive a direct synaptic input from the bipolar cells that are activated by rod photoreceptor cells? Only rod cells respond to dim light, and cats (like most mammals) can see in dim light. Yet the anatomical evidence in cats indicated that their ganglion cells receive little or no direct input from rod-driven bipolar cells.

A major part of the answer lies with the AII amacrine cell. This cell has two apparent functions. Like many other amacrine cells, it transmits a transient response to light to the ganglion cells, thereby sharpening their response to the onset of stimulation. But it also serves to connect rod-activated bipolar cells to ganglion cells. By doing so it allows the ganglion cells to function under both bright and dim light conditions. In fact, the AII amacrine cell by virtue of these connections becomes part of the retina's through pathway. The flow of information is from rod photoreceptor to bipolar to AII amacrine to ganglion cell. It makes sense that the AII amacrine cells are small and densely packed: they thereby keep the level of acuity high along that crucial path.

The third cell, like the first, is identified by its neurotransmitter, in this case dopamine. Tauchi and I found we could use the same kind of fluores-

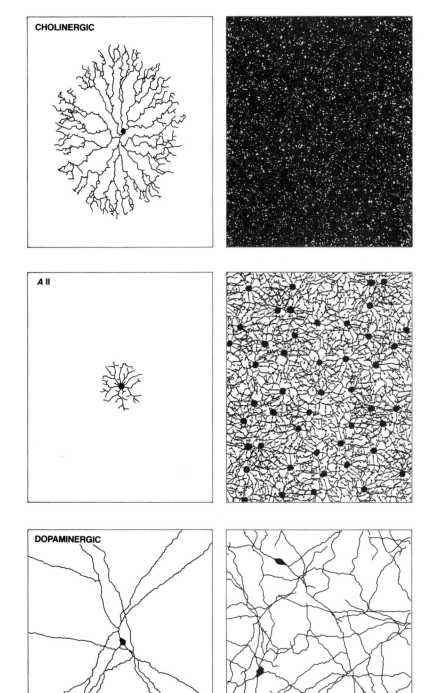

Figure 99 MOSAICS of different amacrine cells cover the retina differently. Three cell types are shown in flat view. Individual cells are at the left; drawings at the right show an approximation of the mosaic that would result if all the cells of a class were stained simultaneously. Cholinergic cells are numerous and their branching dendrites form an almost uninterrupted meshwork (*top*). The mosaic of AII cells is sparser (*middle*), with more space between dendrites. Dopaminergic cells are sparser still (*bottom*).

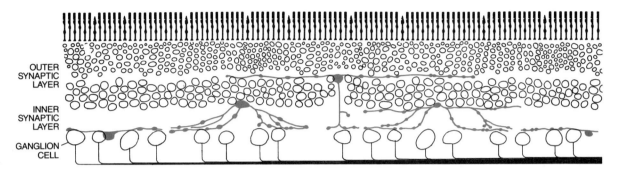

OUTER
SYNAPTIC
LAYER

INNER
SYNAPTIC
LAYER

GANGLION
CELL

Figure 100 INDOLEAMINE-ACCUMULATING CELLS (*color*) come in five shapes. Four are like other amacrine cells; one is unusual, bridging between the outer and inner synaptic layers. They all send processes to the lowest level of the inner synaptic layer, where most or all of them synapse with rod-driven bipolar cells. They appear to provide five pathways to a common end point.

cent injection method on these cells as on the cholinergic cells. What is notable about the dopaminergic cells is their scarcity in the retina. To give an example, the rabbit retina incorporates (in round numbers) some 350,000 ganglion cells and 300,000 cholinergic amacrine cells but only some 8,500 dopaminergic amacrine cells. Furthermore, the dendrites of the dopamine-containing cells are few and are thinly branched, resulting in a mosaic that is full of spaces, not densely packed as in the case of the other amacrine cells discussed here.

Although the precise function of the dopaminergic cells is not known, the loose mosaic does clearly suggest that these cells are not involved in activities that require a high degree of spatial resolution. Whereas the exceptionally densely packed mosaic of the cholinergic amacrine cell makes possible the exact resolution of a small spot crossing the retina, in the dopaminergic cells a small spot would often fall on one of the holes in the mosaic. In other words, it is unlikely that the dopaminergic cell controls any of the obvious features of the ganglion cell's receptive fields. Electron microscope observations by John E. Dowling and Ehinger, working at Harvard, show that dopaminergic cells have synapses only with other amacrine cells. They have no direct connection to the retina's primary through pathway. Moreover, electrophysiological experiments indicate that the dopaminergic cells affect the activity of ganglion cells in a vague way that is hard to define. One possibility is that they have some rather diffuse function, such as mediating the overall excitability of the inner retinal neurons.

The last amacrine cell to be discussed is distinguished experimentally by its accumulation of chemical analogues of the neurotransmitter serotonin. Because serotonin and the analogues are indoleamines, the cells are termed "indoleamine-accumulating." After labeling the retina with a fluorescent serotonin analogue, 5,7-dihydroxytryptamine, Julie H. Sandell (a postdoctoral student) and I were able to examine these cells and study their morphology.

We found that this class of amacrine cells can be subdivided into five distinct morphological types. They have so many features in common, however, that it is best to consider them a family of cells rather than functionally independent cell types. There are many reasons for this. First, their dendrites share a family resemblance in size, shape and branching pattern that sets them apart from the dendrites of other amacrine cells. Second, they transport and accumulate the same serotonin and analogue. Finally, and most important, their dendrites all participate in a dense plexus, or network, lining the innermost margin of the inner synaptic layer. There the cells make a characteristic synapse, called a reciprocal synapse, with a terminal of the rod-driven bipolar cell.

It is outside the plexus that the differences among these cells manifest themselves, and this is reflected in their synaptic connections and their overall shapes. Because the indoleamine-accumulating cells branch extensively and are in contact with many if not all rod-driven bipolar cells, they are thought to have a major influence on the pathway by which dim light passes through the retina. The logical conclusion is that the five indoleamine-accumulating

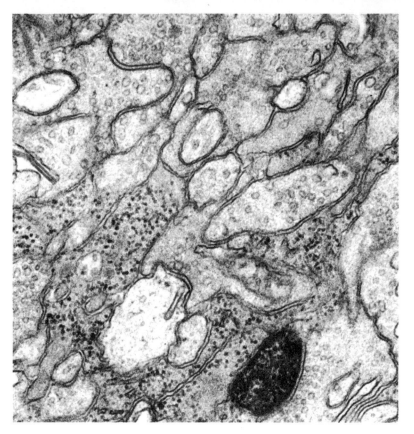

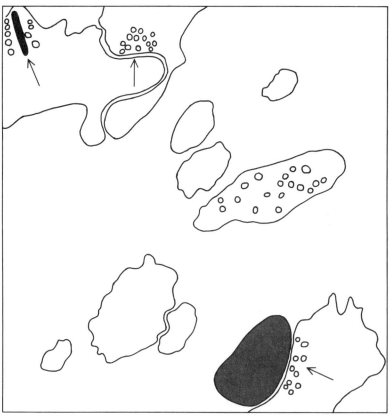

Figure 101 INNER SYNAPTIC LAYER is enlarged some 45,000 diameters in the micrograph (*top*). The dendrites of a number of neurons can be seen; a few of them are indicated on the map (*bottom*). The dark material in one dendrite identifies the dendrite as that of an indoleamine-accumulating cell. Vesicles (*small circles*) containing neurotransmitters are seen at synapses (*arrows*). (Micrograph by R. F. Dacheux and E. Raviola of the Harvard Medical School.)

cells represent five different pathways by which other retinal neurons can interact with rod bipolar cells.

As this small sample of the amacrine cells makes plain, the retina contains a great deal of extremely sophisticated circuitry. In fact, the complexity of the retina is dismaying even to neurobiologists. "The retina is supposed to be a simple system," colleagues typically complain. "How can it be more complicated than other brain structures?" To tease them one can respond that the retina seems complicated only because more is known about it. (The unspoken fear, of course, is that the retina is not notably complicated; if a structure thought to be a prototype of simplicity is really this intricate, what must the cerebral cortex be like?) There are more serious answers, however.

The first answer is that the overall task of the retina, the conversion of light signals into meaningful trains of nerve impulses, demands complex machinery. This article has addressed only one aspect of the retina's coding of visual input: the organization of two kinds of ganglion cell receptive fields. I have completely omitted, for example, the retina's remarkable ability to alter its own sensitivity levels. It does so through internal adjustments in responsiveness, which take place at every stage in the retinal hierarchy. It is these adjustments that enable most mammals to see effectively in both sunlight and starlight, a 10-billionfold range in light intensity. Retinas are also able to transmit information to the brain about the wavelengths of the light they receive, enabling human beings and some other vertebrates to see colors. Given the sophisticated tasks accomplished by the retina, it makes sense that its wiring is complicated.

A second answer is that sophisticated circuitry may be required even for what seem to be straightforward tasks. There was no way to predict, for example, that the rod bipolar cells would be found not to synapse directly with ganglion cells. Making the connection by way of the AII amacrine cells seems illogical. Not only is it an indirect mode of communication but also it adds lateral spread (admittedly a small one) to the visual pathway and thereby threatens visual acuity. If cone bipolar cells make contact with ganglion cells directly, why should rod cells be any different? The only conclusion to be drawn is that the presence of AII amacrine cells solves some problem we are not even aware of yet.

The third and perhaps the best answer is that the retina packages a lot of complexity within a small area. All parts of the central nervous system operate under constraints of space, but rarely is space as limited as it is in the retina. There are two reasons for this: retinal cells must be packed together very tightly to maximize visual acuity, and the retina must be very thin (in the rabbit about a tenth of a millimeter) so that light can penetrate to the rods and cones. One square millimeter of the rabbit's central retina overlies 9.4 linear meters of cholinergic cell dendrites alone. Add to this the dendrites of all the other neurons in the retina, and the density of cell processes is staggering. It is not surprising, then, that retinal neurons are smaller than most other neurons. If their cell bodies were the same size as those of the human brain, the human eye would be almost the size of a tangerine. In short, the retina is a triumph of miniaturization.

Research on the architecture of the retina is about to enter a new and promising phase: the reconstruction in three dimensions of functionally related groups of neurons. The methods we have developed for revealing the shapes of retinal neurons can readily be combined with electron microscopy. They simplify the electron microscopist's task by providing a guide for following individual dendrites through the thickets of each synaptic layer. Furthermore, the same miniaturization that usually presents a barrier to the investigation of retinal cells becomes an advantage when one attempts three-dimensional reconstruction. The close packing of retinal cells makes it easier to examine entire retinal circuits in electron micrographs of serial tissue sections and then to reconstruct the circuitry.

Although this kind of investigation is now in its infancy, the value of space-filling models is clear. Such neural reconstructions are the ultimate description of the architecture and interconnections of retinal cells. Other kinds of inquiry will be necessary before one can say how those structures function electrically and chemically. When the structures are known, however, the work begun by Ramón y Cajal nearly a century ago will have been completed.

Transplantation in the Central Nervous System

Transplanted embryonic neurons can establish functional connections in the adult brain and spinal cord, long believed to be immutable in mammals. Such grafts might reverse damage from disease or injury.

. . .

Alan Fine

August, 1986

Can damage done to the brain or the spinal cord by disease or injury be repaired? Neurons, or nerve cells, cannot regenerate in adult mammals. The great majority of them are in place by the end of infancy, and in primates, including human beings, the development of the nervous system is complete by puberty. Axons, the threadlike extensions of nerve cells along which messages travel, can regrow after damage—a capacity underlying the slow return of feeling and movement after certain injuries—but they generally do so only in peripheral nerves. In the brain or spinal cord a damaged pathway rarely re-forms.

Even though the mammalian central nervous system (the brain and spinal cord) shows little capacity on its own for regeneration, over the past decade it has been found capable of sustaining new growth of another kind. In a series of experiments done mainly in rats, other investigators and I have shown that grafts of embryonic brain tissue can be anatomically and functionally incorporated into the adult central nervous system. The interactions of grafts and their host nervous system have revealed much about the factors governing development and regeneration in the central nervous system. The success of certain transplantation experiments has also suggested ways to treat currently incurable disorders, such as Parkinson's disease and Alzheimer's disease, in which parts of the central nervous system degenerate.

The work of the past decade was foreshadowed by a number of earlier efforts. In 1890 W. Gilman Thompson of New York University Medical College tried to transplant pieces of cerebral cortex (the outer layer of the brain) from adult cats to dogs. No neurons survived these procedures or similar manipulations by other workers over the next 15 years. Elizabeth Hopkins Dunn, a physician working as a research assistant at the University of Chicago, guessed that although adult brain tissue did not stand up to the rigors of transplantation, immature tissue might. In work done in 1903 (but not reported

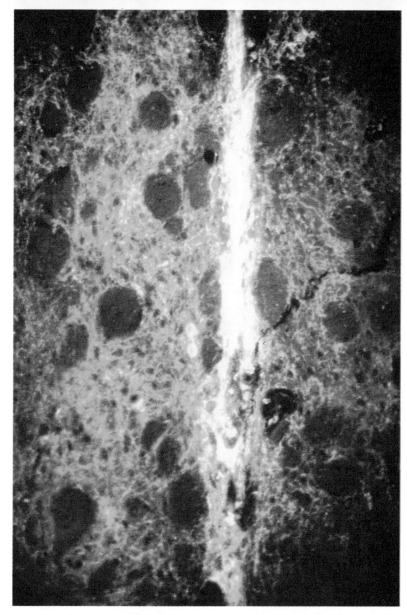

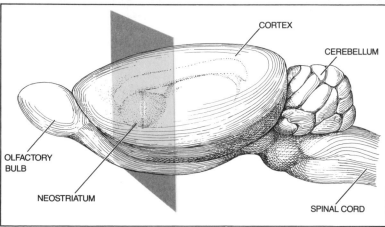

CORTEX

CEREBELLUM

OLFACTORY
BULB

NEOSTRIATUM

SPINAL CORD

Figure 102 YELLOW FLUORES-
CENCE marks nerve cells transplanted into a rat brain. Nerve
fibers containing dopamine were
eliminated from the neostriatum
in order to induce an analogue of
Parkinson's disease. Neurons that
synthesize dopamine were taken
from a rat embryo and injected
into the neostriatum. Six months
later a cross section of the host
brain was treated with formalde-
hyde vapor, which combines with
dopamine to form a fluorescent
compound. Fluorescence at and
around the implant shows the
transplanted neurons had survived, had sent fibers into the
neostriatum and had continued to
make dopamine. (Image from A.
Björklund of the University of
Lund.)

until 1917) she exchanged fragments of cortex between 10-day-old rats. In 10 percent of the cases she found surviving neurons in the grafts three months after surgery.

In addition to establishing the fact that immature neural tissue has a better chance of surviving in another brain than adult tissue has, Dunn noticed that the surviving grafts in most cases were those that were richly supplied with new blood vessels. Such transplants had been placed in the ventricles, or fluid-filled spaces, of the host brain, in contact with choroid plexus, the highly vascular membrane that lines the ventricles. In 1940 W. E. Le Gros Clark of the University of Oxford confirmed the importance of immaturity and a rich blood supply for the survival of transplanted neurons. He successfully transferred pieces of cortex from rabbit embryos to the lateral ventricles in six-week-old rabbits. Although the neurons were immature when they were grafted, four weeks later he found that many of them had completed their development.

Many investigators were skeptical about these early results, and the work was not pursued. Current interest in transplantation in the mammalian central nervous system dates from 1971, when Gopal D. Das, Joseph Altman and their students at Purdue University demonstrated beyond doubt that transplanted immature neurons can survive and mature. These workers injected radioactively labeled thymidine, one of the building blocks of DNA, into seven-day-old rats, where the compound was incorporated into the genetic material of newborn cells, including neurons. Das and Altman then transplanted fragments of the cerebellum (a convoluted structure at the back of the brain) from the injected animals to the matching site in untreated animals. Two weeks later they took sections of the host cerebellum and coated them with photographic emulsion. Radioactivity in the sections exposed the emulsion, indicating that transplanted neurons had survived.

In later experiments Das and Altman established the general principle that embryonic brain tissue transplanted during the period when neurons multiply and migrate, before they extend their filamentous axons and dendrites, has the best chance of survival. Because different parts of the brain develop at different rates, the optimum age of the donor animal varies according to the kind of graft that is intended. The age of the host animal has far less bearing on the survival of transplanted tissue than do factors such as the physical stability of the implant and the blood supply available to the graft.

A condition that is now known to have less effect on transplant survival than had been expected is the degree of kinship between the donor and the host animal. In other kinds of graft immunologic rejection swiftly ensues if the donor and the host are not closely related. Accordingly most of the early transplantation experiments were done in closely related or genetically identical animals. It was later learned that immunologic rejection of a graft in the central nervous system may not occur even when the donor and the host animal are genetically different. Indeed, transplants to the central nervous system can succeed between animals of different species, particularly when the host animal has been treated with an immunosuppressive drug such as cyclosporin.

The observation that the brain is an "immunologically privileged" site for transplantation did not originate with grafts of neurons. Earlier work had shown that grafted skin and tumor tissue could survive in the brain even in an animal that promptly rejected similar grafts to its skin. It is thought that because the brain lacks lymphatic vessels and lymph nodes, from which many of the cells of the immune system are deployed, and because the walls of blood vessels in the central nervous system are specialized to create a "blood-brain barrier," the access of the immune system to foreign tissue in the brain is limited.

In the case of neuronal transplants the lack of rejection may also reflect the characteristics of nerve cells proper. On their surface most cells bear large molecules known as class I major histocompatibility antigens. The antigens are distinctive in each animal; they are the molecules the immune system recognizes as foreign when it rejects grafted tissue. It is now known that those antigens are normally rare or absent on most neurons.

The routine survival of transplanted neural tissue opens the way to study of its interaction with the host. One line of inquiry to which the technique has been applied is the identification of factors governing the response of the central nervous system to injury. Transplants can serve to alter conditions in a traumatized brain or spinal cord, making it possible to gauge the relation of a given factor to the limited regenerative capacity of central neurons.

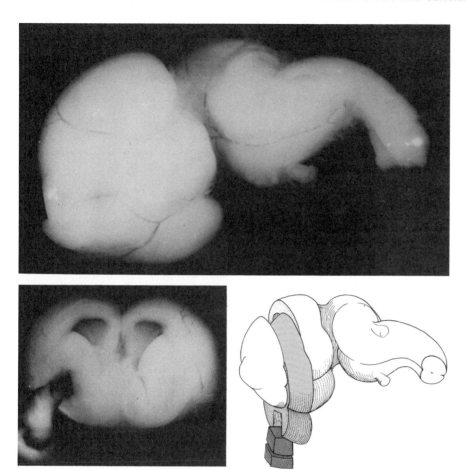

Figure 103 EMBRYONIC RAT BRAIN (*top*), seen from below is from a 17-day embryo (rat pups are born at about 22 days), at which stage the neurons are still multiplying and migrating through the brain. When transplanted to an adult brain, such neurons can mature and send axons into host tissue. The inner piece of tissue dissected from a slice of embryonic brain (*left*) contains cells that are the precursors of the nucleus basalis. Such cells, implanted into an adult rat, can reverse a defect that simulates a feature of Alzheimer's disease. The diagram (*right*) shows the orientation of the slice in the intact brain.

It was known, for example, that the difference between the regenerative capacity of axons in peripheral nerves and that of axons in the central nervous system is correlated with a difference in their glial cells. Those cells surround the axons and can myelinate them, that is, encase the fibers in a sheath of fatty, electrically insulating material. Peripheral nerves are myelinated by Schwann cells; the myelinating cells in the brain and spinal cord are oligodendrocytes.

Studies of sensory neurons, which have both a central and a peripheral fiber, suggest glial cells influence regeneration. From a site just outside the spinal cord a sensory nerve cell extends one fiber to a sensory structure in the periphery of the body and another into the spinal cord. The peripheral fiber, which is myelinated only by Schwann cells, ordinarily regenerates after damage. The great Spanish neuroanatomist Santiago Ramón y Cajal noticed 60 years ago that if the central fiber is crushed, it will regrow only to the point where it enters the spinal cord and oligodendrocytes replace Schwann cells.

A number of workers have suggested that either oligodendrocytes secrete a substance inhibiting axon growth or Schwann cells somehow stimulate axons to grow. Several ways in which Schwann cells might promote fiber growth have already been identified. They secrete proteins such as laminin that have been found in culture to promote the growth of axons and their adhesion to a surface. In response to peripheral-nerve injury Schwann cells may also produce nerve growth factor, a well-studied substance that fosters survival and fiber growth in certain peripheral nerve cells.

In 1977 Carl C. Kao and his collaborators at Georgetown University tested the possibility that peripheral glia might support the regeneration of damaged fibers in the central nervous system. They used delicate surgical techniques to splice lengths of sciatic nerve (a major peripheral nerve) into gaps made by removing a section of the spinal cord in rats. Within weeks, the workers found, the graft and the cord healed to form a smooth, scar-free union, and some fibers seemed to have grown from the spinal cord into the peripheral-nerve segment.

Albert J. Aguayo, Peter M. Richardson and their colleagues at the Montreal General Hospital and McGill University have confirmed and extended those findings. A month after replacing lengths of spinal cord with segments of sciatic nerve from the same rats, they examined the cords under both the light and the electron microscope and noted many fibers growing into the grafts. After three months, by injecting minute quantities of the enzyme horseradish peroxidase into the spinal cord adjacent to the graft, the workers were able to demonstrate that some of the regenerating fibers had succeeded in growing all the way through the graft, bridging the severed ends of the cord.

Horseradish peroxidase is taken up by nerve terminals and carried back along the axons to the cell bodies; incubation in a solution that is chemically altered by the enzyme stains cell bodies whose axons have transported it. In the grafted rats staining appeared in spinal neurons on the other side of the graft from the injection site; their fibers must have grown through the segment of peripheral nerve. In later work Aguayo and his colleagues found that although the regenerating fibers can span grafts several centimeters long, they continue

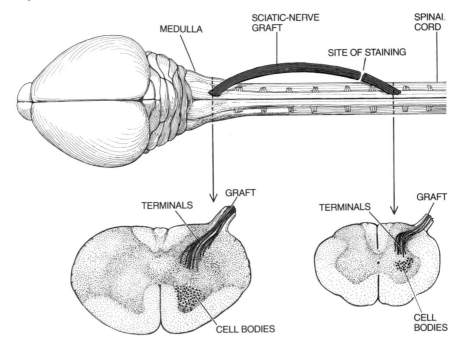

Figure 104 BRIDGE OF PERIPHERAL NERVE grafted into rat central nervous system to study the nerve's effect on axon growth. One end of a sciatic nerve segment was inserted into the medulla and the other end into the spinal cord. After six months the graft was severed and a stain applied to the cut surfaces; cross sections of the medulla and spinal cord at each end of the graft were then examined. Both sites contained stained cell bodies; the sections revealed stained fibers coursing from the nerve segment into the adjacent host tissue. Evidently neurons in both the medulla and spinal cord had sent fibers all the way through the nerve graft.

into the spinal cord beyond the graft for only a few millimeters at most.

Transplantation experiments thus can shed light on the differing regenerative capacities of the peripheral and central nervous systems. A similar contrast in the ability to regenerate and reestablish connections is evident between the embryonic brain, which undergoes extensive changes as it develops and often can recover from injury, and the adult brain. By transplanting pieces of embryonic rat brain to injured adult brains Anders Björklund and Ulf Stenevi of the University of Lund and Lawrence F. Kromer, then at the University of California at San Diego Medical Center, identified one possible basis of the difference.

Before doing the transplants the investigators severed a band of nerve fibers known as the fimbria at its entrance to the hippocampus, a folded and curved sheet of evolutionarily ancient cortex that in human beings plays a role in memory and emotion. The fimbria includes fibers arising in two structures of the forebrain, the medial septal nucleus and the diagonal band nucleus. The fibers contain the neurotransmitter acetylcholine, one of the brain's chemical messengers. Cutting the fimbria eliminates acetylcholine and its synthesizing enzyme, choline acetyltransferase, permanently from most of the upper hippocampus.

When the workers transplanted a piece of embryonic rat hippocampus into the gap in the fimbria, the cholinergic (acetylcholine-releasing) fibers grew through the graft and into the host hippocampus. Six months later choline acetyltransferase in the hippocampus adjacent to the graft was restored to as much as 50 percent of its normal level. Similar experiments using other parts of the embryonic brain have indicated that embryonic tissue can act as a bridge for the growth of axons in the central nervous system, provided the grafted tissue is the normal target of the axons. The results suggest embryonic brain structures may produce specific neurotrophic factors (substances that stimulate the growth of nerve cells and fibers) that guide developing fibers to their targets. Alternatively, grafted embryonic tissue may somehow induce the host brain to produce such factors.

That the adult brain can secrete neurotrophic factors under certain conditions is borne out by observations made by Ellen R. Lewis and Carl W. Cotman at the University of California at Irvine in 1982. They noted that embryonic brain tissue transplanted to cavities made in the brain of adult rats survived better in cavities formed between three and six days before the implant than in cavities made earlier or more recently. During that interval, the investigators surmised, some neurotrophic factor made or accumulated by the central nervous system following an injury must reach its greatest concentration.

Together with Manuel Nieto-Sampedro and other colleagues, the Irvine workers demonstrated the presence of such a factor by collecting fluid from the cavities and adding it to neurons in culture. The fluid extended the survival of the neurons, and the effect was greatest when the cavity was between three and six days old. Such a factor might act as an analogue of nerve growth factor and stimulate the limited fiber growth seen after certain injuries to the central nervous system.

In addition to pointing to influences on the overall extent of fiber growth, the fate of neural transplants hints at factors that control the establishment of specific patterns of connections in the brain. In contrast to the normal inability of adult neurons to grow new fibers or regenerate injured ones, grafted embryonic neurons are able to extend fibers into the host brain routinely. This growth is not indiscriminate. The normal anatomical relation of the grafted and the host tissue and the existing innervation of the host structures both influence the extent and pattern of fiber growth.

Fibers extending from grafted tissue are most likely to grow into the structures normally innervated by that tissue. Björklund, Stenevi and their co-workers transplanted embryonic neurons to the cortex of adult rats and also to the neostriatum, a region that lies under the cortex in the forebrain and is related to movement. The neurons were taken from the substantia nigra, a midbrain structure that sends many fibers containing the neurotransmitter dopamine to the neostriatum but very few to the cortex. The cells survived in both places but sent out appreciable numbers of fibers only in the neostriatum, normally their principal target.

Raymond D. Lund, then at the Medical University of South Carolina, and his students C. B. Jaeger and Steven C. and Linda Kirschen McLoon made detailed observations about the specificity with which grafts interact with host brains. They transplanted embryonic retinas to the brains of newborn

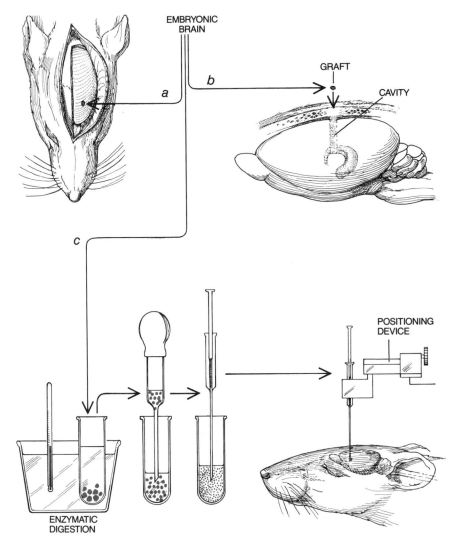

Figure 105 SOLID TISSUE dissected from embryonic rat brain can be implanted intact directly into the host brain (*a*). Or, a cavity can be prepared in advance (*b*); blood vessels grow into the walls of the cavity, ensuring a rich blood supply to the graft. In a third approach (*c*), less disruptive of the host brain, embryonic tissue is digested by an enzyme and then passed through a series of progressively finer pipettes to be disrupted. A suspension of single cells results, which can be labeled with a radioactive substance or a dye, stored or manipulated in other ways before being injected into the host rat brain.

and adult rats. In some cases the graft site was the superior colliculus, one of the regions in the brain to which retinal neurons normally send fibers; in others it was the cortex or the cerebellum, areas that receive no retinal inputs. Although the retinas survived in every site, fiber outgrowth ensued only in the superior colliculus. The outgrowing fibers attained the normal targets of retinal fibers in the colliculus and sometimes also followed the normal retinal pathways to more distant targets.

In addition to sending out fibers, tissue transplanted to the brains of newborn rats in some cases also received inputs from the host brain; again the interaction was highly specific. Grafts of retina, which ordinarily is not innervated by other brain structures, received no fiber growth from the host brain. Pieces of embryonic colliculus placed in the superior colliculus of newborn rats, however, not only grew fibers themselves but also became threaded with appropriate inputs from the host retina and cortex. Such results hint at the existence of specific local cues governing fiber growth in the central nervous system.

The finding that grafts send the largest number of fibers into areas of host brain that have been deprived of their normal innervation gives further evidence for specific local influences on fiber growth. In the work of Lund and his colleagues, for example, the retinal grafts generated the most profuse fiber growth when the eye normally sending fibers

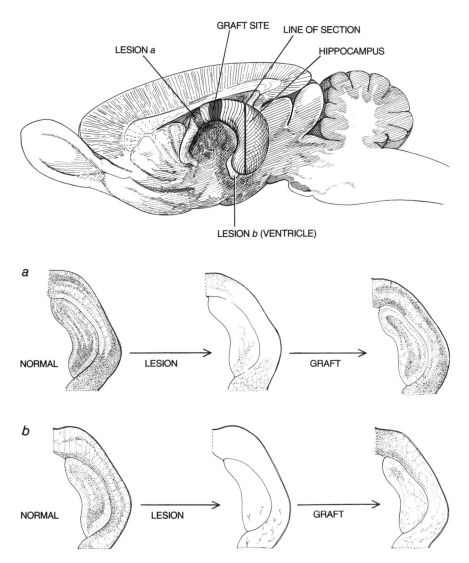

Figure 106 REESTABLISHING NORMAL INNERVATION. Sections in *a* were exposed to a substance that reveals acetylcholine before (*left*) and after (*middle*) the bundle of cholinergic fibers entering the hippocampus was cut (*lesion a*). Four months after embryonic cholinergic neurons were implanted in a denervated hippocampus, a third section (*right*) shows that the grafted cells had reca- pitulated the normal pattern of cholinergic innervation. **Sections in *b* show the normal pattern of noradrenaline-containing fibers (*left*) and their elimination (*middle*) by toxin (*lesion b*). Six months after embryonic noradrenaline tissue was implanted the original innervation pattern was largely reestablished (*right*).**

to the site of the implant had been surgically removed beforehand. Björklund, Stenevi and their coworkers made a similar observation when they transplanted embryonic tissue containing the locus ceruleus, a collection of cells in the brainstem that send fibers containing the neurotransmitter noradrenaline to targets throughout the brain, including the hippocampus. When the tissue was implanted in the hippocampus of adult brains, it extended fibers that recapitulated the pattern of innervation normally established there by the host brain's own locus ceruleus—but only if the pathways from the locus ceruleus had been destroyed before the transplant.

Work not involving transplants has shown that damage to a set of fibers in the central nervous system can result in "collateral axon sprouting": other, healthy fibers extend new branches into the denervated area. The much more luxuriant fiber outgrowth from grafts into denervated brain structures seem to present an analogous case. Taken together, such observations suggest that the growth of nerve fibers from structures in the developing brain as well as from grafts may be regulated by competition either for some scarce diffusible material released by target neurons or for occupancy of particular sites on the target.

S tudies of fiber growth confirm that grafted embryonic tissue can be incorporated anatomically into the host central nervous system. Is the integration functional as well? If it is, could grafts restore normal function to a brain impaired by injury or disease?

Several features of the central nervous system might work in favor of recovery mediated by grafts. For one thing, recovery of function in the central nervous system may not require the precise reconstruction of damaged elements. Many important and complex functions in the brain and spinal cord are performed semiautonomously by discrete structures or assemblies of neurons. To restore a measure of function after an injury that isolates such a structure, it may be sufficient to replace only a few of its inputs.

Over the past 15 years, for example, workers have established that the basic elements of locomotion, such as the rhythmic spinal undulations in fishes and the sequential contractions of the limb muscles that underlie stepping motion in mammals, are generated by groups of neurons in the spinal cord. These "locomotion generators" are subject to several stages of control: they are inhibited by other spinal neurons, which in turn are inhibited by fibers that descend from the brainstem and are thought to release catecholamine neurotransmitters such as noradrenaline and dopamine. Cutting the connection between the brainstem and the spinal cord in a cat gives free rein to the inhibitory spinal neurons and hence paralyzes the animal, but if the cat is injected with L-dopa, a precursor of dopamine, and is supported on a treadmill, it will walk. These observations have suggested that paralysis caused by spinal-cord injury might respond to grafts of embryonic catecholamine neurons into the spinal cord near the locomotion generators, even if the spinal pathways are not repaired.

The spinal cord includes not only long pathways consisting of a single continuous fiber but also pathways made up of multiple short links, in which messages are relayed by a series of neurons. It is therefore conceivable that in a severed spinal cord these multiple-relay pathways, at least, could be mended with transplants of embryonic neurons, which would transmit information across the gap in the pathways.

Neurochemical factors as well as neuroanatomical ones brighten the prospect for graft-mediated recovery of function. The chemistry of the brain changes after it is damaged. These effects have been studied in detail in an experimental analogue of Parkinson's disease. The disease is the result of the degeneration of the dopamine-releasing fibers that extend from the substantia nigra to the neostriatum. The degeneration can be induced in the rat brain by injecting either of the two structures or the bundle of fibers with the substance 6-hydroxydopamine, which selectively destroys neurons, fibers and terminals containing catecholamines such as dopamine.

When the dopamine pathway is destroyed on both sides of the brain, the animal becomes immobile and may die unless it is nursed intensively. A rat injected on only one side no longer responds to sensations on the opposite side of the body, which is controlled by the damaged half of the brain. It develops an asymmetric posture, twisting away from the unresponsive side. When the animal moves, it turns toward its "good" side—the one that received the injection.

If the lesions (the damaged areas) spare more than 5 percent of the dopamine-containing cells or fibers, the animal can recover. Much of the recovery takes place within one or two weeks, far too soon to be the result of regeneration of the damaged fibers or collateral sprouting of other dopaminergic neurons. Experiments done in a number of laboratories, notably that of John F. Marshall of the University of California at Irvine, have identified two kinds of neurochemical changes that take place in the nervous system following injury or damage and may account for the rapid recovery.

One change is an increase in the rate at which surviving fiber terminals synthesize and release neurotransmitter. The other is an increase in the sensitivity of the target neurons to the small amounts of transmitter still being secreted. Such "denervation supersensitivity," which usually results from an increase in the number of receptors for the neurotransmitter on the surface of the target cell, would increase the efficacy of the surviving dopaminergic fibers in the lesioned rats.

Denervation supersensitivity probably accounts for some of the remarkable ability of embryonic neuronal transplants to reverse behavioral abnormalities in animal models of degenerative neurological diseases. The 6-hydroxydopamine model of Parkinson's disease provided the earliest example. Mark J. Perlow, William J. Freed and Richard Jed Wyatt of the National Institute of Mental Health, working with Lars Olson and Åke Seiger of the Karolinska Institute and Barry Hoffer of the University of Colorado Health Sciences Center at Denver, destroyed the substantia nigra on one side of the brain in rats. They then transplanted fragments of embryonic brain containing the precursor cells of the substantia nigra to the lateral ventricle adjacent to the denervated neostriatum.

The movement asymmetries that had resulted from the lesions were reduced after the grafts. Injections of the drug apomorphine confirmed that the transplanted neurons were releasing dopamine. Apomorphine binds to dopamine receptors and activates them. Its effect yields a measure of denervation supersensitivity: neurons that lack their usual input of dopamine will be unusually sensitive to apomorphine. Thus injecting it into the neostriatum of a lesioned rat causes the rat to reverse its turning and twist away from the lesion: the neostriatum on the damaged side in effect overreacts to the drug. Because some dopamine input to the neostriatum had been restored by the grafts, the grafted rats'

response to apomorphine was only half as great as the response of lesioned rats that had not received the grafts, and the reduction lasted for the length of the experiment: more than six months (see Figure 107).

Freed and Wyatt have found that implants of cells from the adrenal gland, a hormone-secreting structure above the kidney, can also reverse some of the effects of 6-hydroxydopamine injection. The cells, taken from the medulla, or central part, of the gland, normally produce adrenaline, a hormone derived from dopamine. When medullary cells are removed from the gland, they may secrete dopamine instead. Like the neuronal transplants, the cells were placed in the lateral ventricle, and they reduced the rats' movement asymmetry but not their sensory abnormalities. Grafts of tissue from embryonic substantia nigra into sites within or very near the neostriatum, done by Björklund and Stenevi, in collaboration with Susan D. Iversen and Stephen B. Dunnett of the University of Cambridge, reduced or abolished the rats' movement disorder and also eliminated the animals' sensory asymmetry altogether.

Experimental models of Alzheimer's disease offer another striking example of transplant-mediated recovery. The progressive loss of memory and other higher mental functions in Alzheimer's disease is associated with widespread degeneration of neurons and neurochemical abnormalities, notably a depletion of acetylcholine in the hippocampus and much of the cortex. Depriving the rat hippocampus of its main acetylcholine input by cutting the fimbria has been found in many laboratories to impair certain kinds of learning, in particular the spatial kind that is needed to learn a maze.

Björklund and his co-workers, including Fred H. Gage, transplanted solid pieces of tissue from the forebrain structures that normally supply the hippocampus with acetylcholine into the cut fimbria of rats; in other rats the workers introduced the tissue directly into the denervated hippocampus in the form of disaggregated cells. The grafts improved the animals' ability to learn a maze — an effect that was most pronounced when the animals were also injected with physostigmine, a drug that blocks the degradation of acetylcholine and thereby enhances its effects.

The cerebral cortex, which is also affected in Alzheimer's disease, gets its input of acetylcholine from the nucleus basalis of Meynert, a cluster of cells at

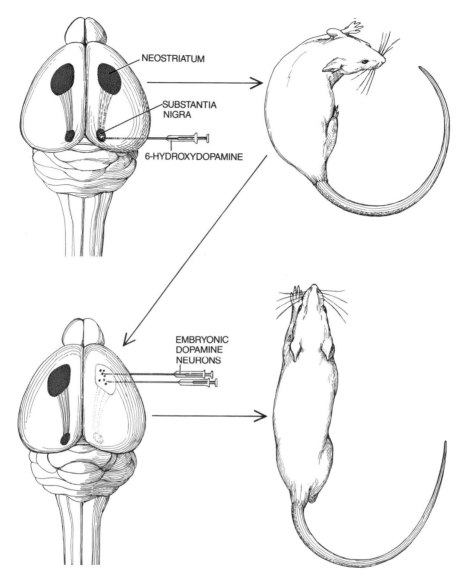

Figure 107 EXPERIMENTAL PARKINSON'S DISEASE induced in a rat. An injection of 6-hydroxydopamine destroys the substantia nigra, which sends dopamine-containing fibers to the neostriatum. Bilateral injections severely debilitate the animal, but if injected on one side only, the rat develops an asymmetry of posture and movement: it turns spontaneously toward the injected side. Transplantation of dopamine-producing neurons from rat embryos to the denervated neostriatum eliminates the movement asymmetry for at least six months.

the base of the forebrain. Those cells degenerate in Alzheimer's disease. To simulate this feature of the disease my colleagues, including Dunnett and Guy Toniolo of the University of Strasbourg, and I injected the region of the nucleus basalis on one side of the rat brain with the toxin ibotenic acid. The toxin, which destroys neurons but spares nerve fibers passing through the injected area, permanently eliminates almost all the acetylcholine input from the nucleus basalis to the cortex on the injected side. Certain sensory and movement asymmetries result from the injection, along with serious

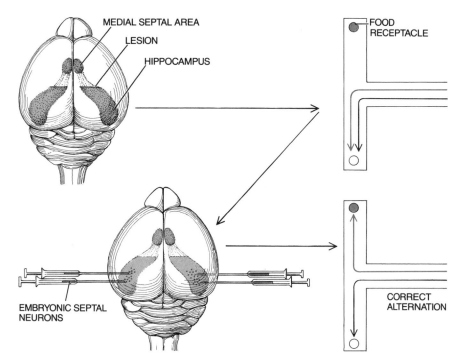

Figure 108 FEATURE OF ALZHEIMER'S DISEASE, a loss of acetylcholine from the hippocampus, can be simulated in the rat by cutting the cholinergic fibers leading from the medial septal area to the hippocampus. Normal rats can be trained with food rewards to enter opposite arms of a T-maze in strict alternation, but rats with cut fibers do not learn to alternate. Instead they reenter the same side several times in a row. When embryonic neurons taken from the medial septal area are injected into the hippocampus of such rats, they can again learn to alternate sides.

impairment of the rat's ability to learn and remember simple tasks, such as avoiding the dark chamber in a two-chamber maze or finding a submerged platform in a pool of water.

Because the neurons of the nucleus basalis are interspersed among various other brain structures, the ibotenic acid inevitably destroys a range of cells that send fibers to parts of the brain other than the cortex. Consequently it is unclear whether the behavioral abnormalities of injected rats stem only from the destruction of the cholinergic pathways from the nucleus basalis to the cortex or also reflect damage to other pathways. The ability of transplants of embryonic nucleus basalis to reverse the abnormalities, we thought, would resolve that question and thereby clarify the role of the nucleus basalis in normal functioning.

We found that grafts of cells taken from the precursor region of the nucleus basalis in rat embryos and implanted directly into the denervated cortex of the toxin-injected rats restored their spatial memory to normal, although the grafted rats still learned their tasks more slowly than normal rats did. The grafts also corrected some of the movement asymmetries but did not reverse the sensory deficits. Control transplants of cells from embryonic hippocampus, which lack acetylcholine, were entirely without effect.

As well as suggesting that transplants may be able to reverse Alzheimer's-like deficits, the outcome also confirms that the cholinergic pathways from the nucleus basalis to the cortex play a role in the spatial memory that was impaired in lesioned rats. Transplantation could be applied in much the same way to the analysis of functional neuroanatomy throughout the central nervous system. Where it is difficult to remove only part of a widely projecting pathway or a complex structure in order to investigate function in detail, it may be possible to achieve the same end by destroying the entire structure or pathway and then reconstructing with grafted tissue the part that is of interest.

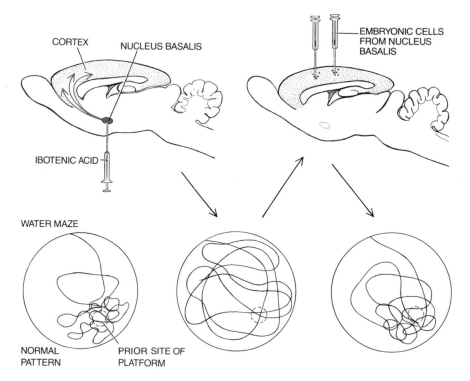

CORTEX NUCLEUS BASALIS

EMBRYONIC CELLS FROM NUCLEUS BASALIS

IBOTENIC ACID

WATER MAZE

NORMAL PATTERN

PRIOR SITE OF PLATFORM

Figure 109 ANOTHER FEATURE OF ALZHEIMER'S, the depletion of acetylcholine in the cortex, is simulated by an injection of ibotenic acid that destroys the large cells of the nucleus basalis, which send cholinergic fibers to the cortex. A normal rat, trained to find a submerged platform, will swim over the site as though searching for the plat- form even if it is removed. The path of an injected rat suggests the animal does not remember the platform's original position. After transplanting embryonic cells from the nucleus basalis to the cortex, such a rat can again be trained to remember the site.

Denervation supersensitivity by itself is not enough to account for the substantial behavioral effects of neuronal grafts. In the normal brain many nerve cells relay precisely patterned messages in response to appropriate inputs from other neurons. Grafted neurons often are transplanted not to their normal site but to a distant target, and it is not known whether they establish a normal pattern of synapses: the zones of communication with target neurons at which most neurons release neurotransmitter. If transplanted neurons do not communicate specifically with host neurons, how might transplants restore any impaired behavior at all?

Their efficacy suggests that dopamine, acetylcholine and presumably other neurotransmitters often act not to relay critically patterned messages but to modulate the general level or nature of target cells' activity or their response to other inputs. Given those conditions a neurotransmitter might be effec-

tive even if its release is largely unregulated and it reaches its target by gradual diffusion.

In contrast to neurotransmitters, the hormones that are secreted by certain structures in the brain normally travel considerable distances to their targets, and their release may be regulated not by signals from adjacent cells but by diffusible factors carried in the blood or released by other brain structures. Neuroendocrine diseases, the result of deficiencies in particular brain hormones, are therefore promising candidates for treatment with neural grafts. The first such disease in which the technique has been tried in the laboratory is diabetes insipidus. It is characterized by excessive thirst and urination. The symptoms reflect a lack of vasopressin, a hormone that regulates fluid balance and blood pressure by directing the kidney to concentrate urine and causing the peripheral blood vessels to constrict.

The hormone, which also seems to exert behavioral effects in the brain, is made by neurons in the front of the hypothalamus, a brain structure that regulates many physiological functions. The neurons send axons into the posterior part of the pituitary gland, where the vasopressin is released. Diabetes insipidus in humans almost always results from tumors or trauma affecting the pituitary, but a strain of laboratory rats displays an inherited form of the disease. They are born without the vasopressin-producing neurons.

Don M. Gash and John R. Sladek, Jr., of the University of Rochester School of Medicine and Dentistry transplanted fragments of embryonic hypothalamus to a brain ventricle in affected rats. In about 25 percent of the cases the workers observed a sustained improvement in fluid balance: water intake declined and urine became concentrated. Six months after the transplantation the workers found many vasopressin-containing neurons surviving within the grafts.

The neuroendocrine disease known as hypogonadotrophic hypogonadism or Kallmann's syndrome also has a laboratory model. The disease, an inherited condition associated with the X sex chromosome, prevents sexual maturation in boys. The missing hormone is gonadotropin-releasing hormone (GnRH). Made in the hypothalamus, GnRH causes the pituitary to secrete other hormones, which in turn bring about the maturation of the testes and the production of testosterone, the male sex hormone.

The same condition occurs in certain mutant mice. The late Dorothy T. Krieger, working with Perlow and Marie J. Gibson of the Mount Sinai School of Medicine in New York, Harry M. Charlton of the University of Oxford and other investigators, treated hypogonadal mice by transplanting GnRH-containing neurons from embryos to a cerebral ventricle, close to the cells' normal position in the hypothalamus. Within two months the recipients' testes had partially matured and were making normal sperm. A later examination of the mouse brains showed a luxuriant growth of fibers extending from the transplanted neurons toward their normal targets: specialized capillaries that transport GnRH to the pituitary gland.

The root of a hormonal deficiency need not lie within the brain for an intracerebral transplant to have potential value. Efforts to treat endocrine disorders such as diabetes mellitus by transplanting hormone-secreting tissue to other sites in experimental animals or human patients fail unless the subjects are given strong immunosuppressive drug treatment to prevent graft rejection. Implanted in the immunologically privileged confines of the brain, however, such tissue might survive and function. The circulating chemical stimuli that trigger hormone secretion are present in the cerebrospinal fluid that fills the brain ventricles, and secreted hormones could return to the circulatory system by way of the special cellular membranes that transport minute droplets of cerebrospinal fluid to the blood.

The idea was tested more than 40 years ago by Charles M. Pomerat and his co-workers at the University of Alabama. They transplanted tissue from the adrenal gland of newborn rats to the brain of adult rats whose adrenals had been removed. The grafted tissue survived and matured, and for more than eight months it corrected the hormonal deficiencies brought on by the glands' removal.

Recently I and, independently, Wah Jun Tze and Joseph Tai of the University of British Columbia reversed chemically induced diabetes mellitus in rats by transplanting insulin-secreting cells from the pancreas of other rats to the brain of the diabetic animals. Tze and Tai have shown that such transplants are also effective in the spontaneously occurring diabetes, found in a particular rat strain, that is considered the closest animal analogue of human juvenile-onset, insulin-dependent diabetes.

As understanding grows of the biology of transplants in the mammalian central nervous system, their potential to halt its deterioration or restore lost capacities will be tested in a growing number of disorders. Together with Francesco Scaravilli of the National Hospital in London, for example, I am exploring the possible value of such transplants in the hereditary metabolic defects known as lysosomal storage disorders. Caused by deficiencies in enzymes needed to break down complex molecules within the cell, the disorders often lead to severe neurological deterioration. Appropriate cells transplanted to the brain might replace the missing enzymes and prevent the degeneration. In other work, undertaken with Brian Meldrum and Smita Patel of the Institute of Psychiatry in London and Harry Robertson and Georgia Cottrell of Dalhousie University, I am studying the ability of transplanted inhibitory neurons to suppress epileptic seizures induced experimentally in rats.

The work I have described is only a first step toward the development of reliable therapies for human diseases; the procedures that have succeeded in rats are only now being tried in monkeys, in several laboratories including my own. Yet a sense that it is urgent to attempt neuronal transplants in human beings is widely felt. Many of the human disorders that have been simulated and treated by transplantation in experimental animals are currently incurable. The symptoms of Parkinson's disease can often be alleviated by the drug L-dopa, but the fatal progress of the disease continues. For Alzheimer's disease there is no such palliative. Olson and Seiger, working with Erik-Olof Backlund of the Karolinska Hospital and Institute of Stockholm, have already transplanted cells from the adrenal glands of four patients with severe Parkinson's disease into their brains. None of the patients experienced a significant and lasting recovery, although several of them showed temporary improvements.

For the moment transplantation in the central nervous system of human beings poses an ethical problem. Should experimental procedures that are shown to be successful in imperfect animal models but are unproved in primates and that carry unknown but perhaps serious risks be used to treat patients with progressive and fatal disease? The issue warrants wider consideration than it has received so far. Further ethical questions will arise if experiments in primate models of human disease clearly establish the value of the procedures. Nerve cells derived from certain tumors can be grown in culture and have been transplanted successfully into rodents. The likeliest source of embryonic neurons for transplantation to human beings, however, appears to be tissue from aborted fetuses.

POSTSCRIPT

The field of transplantation in the central nervous system has attracted much attention since 1986. While brain swapping is not about to occur, the field is full of promise (see excellent review articles by Zager and Black, 1988 and Fine and Rubin, 1988). Both peripheral and central nervous tissue have shown a remarkable capacity to incorporate and interact with implanted glial and neuronal tissue. Recent studies suggest that there is a certain degree of integration of graft tissue into the host central nervous system, although the extent of functional reinnervation has not been fully evaluated because of technical limitations. Nevertheless, the mature mammalian brain is able to regenerate specific connections that may be lost because of cell death or injury. However, this requires the presence of undifferentiated replacement cells that are not normally present in the adult central nervous system. Progress has been made regarding the optimal donor tissue for the successful growth and differentiation of neural grafts. Much research remains to be done to determine to what extent intercerebral neural grafting may be a useful therapeutic tool in neurodegenerative diseases or instances of damage to the central nervous system.

The Authors

CHARLES F. STEVENS ("The Neuron") is professor of physiology at the Yale University School of Medicine. He did his undergraduate work in experimental psychology at Harvard University and obtained his M.D. at the Yale School of Medicine and his Ph.D. in biophysics from Rockefeller University in 1964. From 1963 through 1975 he was on the physiology and biophysics faculty of the University of Washington School of Medicine, taking a sabbatical leave during the 1969–70 academic year at the Lorentz Institute for Theoretical Physics at the University of Leiden.

SOLOMON H. SNYDER ("The Molecular Basis of Communication between Cells") is director of the department of neuroscience at the Johns Hopkins University School of Medicine; he is also Distinguished Service Professor of neuroscience, pharmacology and psychiatry. He did his undergraduate work at Georgetown University and earned his medical degree from the Georgetown Medical School in 1962. In 1965 he went to the Johns Hopkins Hospital as an assistant resident in the psychiatry department. A year later he joined the faculty at Johns Hopkins as assistant professor of pharmacology and experimental therapeutics. He was made professor in 1970.

JAMES A. NATHANSON and **PAUL GREENGARD** ("'Second Messengers' in the Brain") are, respectively, at Massachusetts General Hospital in Boston and Rockefeller University. Nathanson attended Trinity College and then studied medicine at Yale, where he became interested in the biochemical approach to brain function and went on to obtain his Ph.D. in neurobiology in Greengard's laboratory. After graduation and a year of medical internship he spent two years at the National Institutes of Health, returning to Yale in 1976 as a resident in neurology. He is also an amateur astronomer and has published a paper on the classification of galaxies. Greengard is professor of pharmacology at Yale. As a 17-year-old in the navy during World War II he was sent to the Massachusetts Institute of Technology to take part in the development of an early-warning system to protect navy ships from Japanese kamikaze planes. After the war he attended Hamilton College and Johns Hopkins University, where his interests evolved from mathematics and physics to neurobiology. After receiving his Ph.D. from Johns Hopkins in 1953 he spent the next five years doing postdoctoral work in England. Greengard became director of the biochemistry department of the Geigy Research Laboratories in 1959 and moved to Yale in 1963.

RODOLFO R. LLINÁS ("Calcium in Synaptic Transmission") is professor and chairman of the department of physiology and biophysics at the New York University Medical Center in New York. Born in Colombia, he received his M.D. from the Pontifical University of Javeriana in 1959. He then moved to Australia as a research scholar at the Australian National University, from which he received his Ph.D. in 1965, and came to the United States as associate professor at the University of Minnesota. From 1966 to 1970 he was on the staff of the Institute for Biomedical Research of the American Medical Association Education and Research Foundation. In 1970 he became professor of physiology and biophysics and head of the division of neurobiology at the University of Iowa; he left Iowa in 1976 to take up his present job at NYU Medical Center. In addition to synaptic transmission Llinás has worked on the electrophysiology of the central nervous system.

ERIC R. KANDEL ("Small Systems of Neurons") is professor of physiology and psychiatry and director of the Division of Neurobiology and Behavior at the Columbia University College of Physicians and Surgeons. He was born in Vienna and came to the U.S. in 1939. He was graduated from Harvard College in 1952 and received his M.D. at the New York University School of Medicine in 1956. After a year of internship at Montefiore Hospital in New York he spent three years as a postdoctoral fellow at the National Institute of Mental Health, working on a cellular study of the hippocampus. He was a resident in psychiatry at the Massachusetts Mental Health Center and the Harvard Medical School from 1960 to 1962 and from 1963 to 1964. In the intervening year he was a National Institutes of Health special fellow at the Institute Marey in Paris. There he began to do research with Ladislav Tauc on the nervous system of *Aplysia*. Kandel has continued to work with *Aplysia* since then. In 1965 he returned to the New York University School of Medicine to develop a neurobiology group, and in 1974 he moved to Columbia.

PAUL H. PATTERSON, DAVID D. POTTER and **EDWIN J. FURSHPAN** ("The Chemical Differentiation of Nerve Cells") are neurobiologists. Patterson is in the Department of Biology at the California Institute of Technology. He acquired his Ph.D. in biochemistry from Johns Hopkins University and joined the faculty of Harvard Medical School in 1970. Potter and Furshpan are on the faculty of Harvard Medical School where they arrived in 1959 following a period as postdoctoral fellows in the department of biophysics at University College London. Potter's doctorate in biology is from Harvard: Furshpan's in animal physiology is from the California Institute of Technology. The work described in their chapter was done with Dennis Bray, Robert B. Campenot, Linda L. Y. Chun, Philippa Claude, Karen Fischer, Story C. Landis, Peter R. Mac-Leish, Doreen McDowell, Richard E. Mains, Colin A. Nurse, Kunihiko Obata, Paul H. O'Lague, Louis F. Reichardt, Patricia A. Walicke and Michel Weber.

DAVID I. GOTTLIEB ("GABAergic Neurons") is professor of neurobiology at the Washington University School of Medicine in St. Louis. He received a bachelor's degree in 1964 at Harpur College of the State University of New York (now SUNY at Binghamton) and a doctorate in neurobiology from Washington University in 1972. To complement his training in neurobiology, he stayed in St. Louis as a postdoctoral fellow in the department of biological chemistry. Gottlieb began work at the medical school in 1976.

FLOYD E. BLOOM ("Neuropeptides") is director of the Arthur Vining Davis Center for Behavioral Neurobiology at the Salk Institute. He is a graduate of Southern Methodist University and the Washington University School of Medicine. Before being appointed to his current position in 1975 he was chief of the laboratory of neuropharmacology and acting director of the Division of Special Mental Health Research Programs of the National Institute of Mental Health at St. Elizabeth's Hospital in Washington. His interest in brain research, he says, "stemmed directly from my medical interest in how the brain monitors and controls blood pressure. The continued pursuit of that simple question has led me to develop and apply a variety of experimental approaches to the task of identifying where and how chemical transmitters communicate messages between nerve cells and how those signals are able to alter behavior."

RICHARD H. MASLAND ("The Functional Architecture of the Retina") is associate professor of physiology at the Harvard Medical School. He received his bachelor's degree at Harvard College and his doctorate from McGill University. Between 1968 and 1971 he was a postdoctoral fellow in neurophysiology at the Stanford Medical School and then moved to Massachusetts General Hospital. He set up his own laboratory there in 1973, and in 1975 he became a member of the faculty at the Harvard Medical School.

ALAN FINE ("Transplantation in the Central Nervous System") works in the Molecular Neurobiology Unit of the Medical Research Council in Cambridge, England. His undergraduate studies were done at Harvard University and were punctuated by years spent in France and Israel. He went on to pursue graduate studies in physiology and veterinary medicine at the University of Pennsylvania. After graduate school he held postdoctoral fellowships at both the National Institute of Mental Health and the Weizmann Institute of Science in Israel. Fine has been in Cambridge since 1983.

Bibliographies

1. The Neuron

Kuffler, Stephen W., and John G. Nicholls. 1976. *From neuron to brain: A cellular approach to the function of the nervous system.* Sinauer Associates.

Steinbach. J. H., and C. F. Stevens. 1976. Neuromuscular transmission. In *Frog neurobiology: A handbook,* ed. R. Llinás and W. Precht. Springer-Verlag.

Hille, Bertil. 1978. Gating in sodium channels of nerve. *Annual Review of Physiology* 38:139–152.

Stevens, Charles F. 1978. Interactions between intrinsic membrane protein and electric field: An approach to studying nerve excitability. *Biophysical Journal* 22 (May): 295–306.

Fambrough, Douglas M. 1979. Control of acetylcholine receptors in skeletal muscle. *Physiological Reviews* 59 (January): 165–227.

Numa, S. 1986. Molecular basis for the function of ionic channels., *Biochemical Society Symposium* 52:119–143.

Cotman C. W., and L. L. Iversen. 1988. Excitatory amino acids in the brain: Focus on NMDA receptors. *Trends in Neuroscience* 10:263–265.

Francioline, F., and A. Petris. 1988. Single channel recording and gating function of ionic channels. *Experientai* 44:183–188.

Kosower, E. M. 1988. A partial structure for the gamma-aminobutyric acid (GABA) receptor is derived from the model for the nicotinic acetylcholine receptor. *FEBS Lett* 231:5–10.

Llinás, R. 1988. The intrinsic electrophysiological properties of mammalian neurons: A new insight into CNS function? *Science* 242 (December 23): 1654–1664.

Neher, E. 1988. The use of the patch clamp technique to study second messenger-mediated cellular events. *Neuroscience* 26:727–734.

2. The Molecular Basis of Communication between Cells

Katzenellenbogen, Benita. 1980. Dynamics of steroid hormone receptor action. *Annual Review of Physiology* 42:17–35.

Krieger, Dorothy T. 1983. Brain peptides: What, where, and why? *Science* 222 (December 2): 975–985.

Sherman, Merry R., and John Stevens. 1984. Structure of mammalian steroid receptors: Evolving concepts and methodological development. *Annual Review of Physiology* 46:83–105.

Snyder, Solomon H. 1984. Drug and neurotransmitter receptors in the brain. *Science* 224 (April 6): 22–31.

Czech, Michael P. 1985. The nature and regulation of the insulin receptor: Structure and function. *Annual Review of Physiology* 47:357–381.

Fujita, T. 1985. Neurosecretion and new aspects of neuroendocronology. *Neurosecretion and the Biology of Neuropeptides, Proceedings of the 9th International Symposium on Neurosecretion,* eds. H. Kobayashi, H. Bern and A. Vrano. Springer-Verlag.

3. "Second Messengers" in the Brain

Robison, Alan, Reginald W. Butcher and Earl W. Sutherland. 1971. *Cyclic AMP.* Academic Press.

Drummond, George I., and Yvonne Ma. 1973. Metabolism and functions of cyclic AMP in nerve. *Progress in Neurobiology* 2:119–176.

Bloom, Floyd E. 1975. The role of cyclic nucleotides in central synaptic function. *Reviews of Physiology, Biochemistry and Pharmacology* 74:1–103.

Greengard, Paul. 1976. Possible role for cyclic nucleotides and phosphorylated membrane proteins in postsynaptic actions of neurotransmitters. *Nature* 260 (March 11): 101–108.

Daly, John W. 1977. *Cyclic Nucleotides in the nervous system.* Plenum Press.

Nathanson, James A. 1977. Cyclic nucleotides and nervous system function. *Physiological Reviews* 57:157–256.

Greengard, Paul. 1987. Neuronal phosphoproteins: Mediators of signal transduction. *Molecular Neurobiology* 1:81–119.

4. Calcium in Synaptic Transmission

Katz, B., and R. Miledi. 1967. A study of synaptic transmission in the absence of nerve impulses. *Journal of Physiology* 192:407–436.

Pumplin, D. W., and T. S. Reese. 1978. Membrane ultrastructure of the giant synapse of the squid *Loligo pealii. Neuroscience* 3 (August): 685–696.

Llinás, R., I. Z. Steinberg and K. Walton. 1981. Presynaptic calcium currents in squid giant synapse. *Biophysical Journal* 33 (March): 289–321.

———. 1981. Relationship between presynaptic calcium current and postsynaptic potential in squid giant synapse. *Biophysical Journal* 33 (March): 323–351.

Llinás, R., M. Sugimori and S. M. Simon. 1982. Transmission by presynaptic spikelike depolarization in the squid giant synapse. *Proceedings of the National Academy of Sciences* 79 (April): 2415–2419.

Chad, J. E., and R. O. Eckert. 1984. Calcium domains associated with individual channels can account for anomalous voltage relations of Ca-dependent responses. *Biophysical Journal* 45:993–999.

Simon, S. M., M. Sugimori and R. Llinás. 1984. Modeling of submembranous calcium-concentration changes and their relation to rate of presynaptic transmitter release in the squid giant synapse. *Biophysical Journal* 45:264a.

Llinás, R., T. McGuinness, C. Leonard, M. Sugimori and P. Greengard. 1985. Intraterminal injection of synapsin I or calcium-calmodulin-dependent protein kinase II alters neurotransmitter release at the squid giant synapse. *Proceedings of the National Academy of Sciences* 82:3035–3039.

Simon, S. M., and R. Llinás. 1985. Compartmentalization of the submembrane calcium activity during calcium influx and its significance in transmitter release. *Biophysical Journal* 48:485–498.

Zucker, R. S., and A. L. Fogelson. 1986. Relationship between transmitter release and presynaptic calcium influx when calcium enters through discrete channels. *Proceedings of the National Academy of Sciences* 83:3032–3036.

Augustine, G. J., M. P. Charlton and S. J. Smith. 1987. Calcium action in synaptic transmitter release. *Annual Review of Neuroscience* 10:633–693.

5. Small Systems of Neurons

Benzer, Seymour. 1973. Genetic dissection of behavior. *Scientific American* 229 (December): 24–37.

Nicholls, John G., and David Van Essen. 1974. *Scientific American* 230 (January): 38–48.

Bentley, David, and Ronald R. Hoy. 1974. The neurobiology of cricket song. *Scientific American* 231 (August): 34–44.

Kandel, Eric R. 1976. *Cellular basis of behavior: An introduction to behavioral neurobiology.* W. H. Freeman and Company.

———. 1979. Cellular insights into behavior and learning. *The Harvey Lectures,* Series 73:29–92.

Goelet, P., V. F. Castellucci, S. Schacher and E. R. Kandel. 1986. The long and the short of long-term memory: A molecular framework. *Nature* 6:322, 419–422.

Neary, J. T. 1986. Modulation of ion channels by Ca2+-activated protein phosphorylation: A biochemical mechanism for associative learning. *Progress in Brain Research* 69:91–106.

6. The Chemical Differentiation of Nerve Cells

O'Lague, Paul H., Kunihiko Obata, Philippa Claude, Edward J. Furshpan and David D. Pottter. 1974. Evidence for cholinergic synapses between dissociated rat sympathetic neurons in cell culture. *Proceedings of the National Academy of Sciences* 71 (September): 3602–3606.

Furshpan, Edward J., Peter R. MacLeish, Paul H. O'Lague and David D. Potter. 1976. Chemical transmission between rat sympathetic neurons and cardiac myocytes developing in microcultures: Evidence for cholinergic, adrenergic, and dual-function neurons. *Proceedings of the National Academy of Sciences* 73 (November): 4225–4229.

Landis, Story C. 1976. Rat sympathetic neurons and cardiac myocytes developing in microcultures: Correlation of the fine structure of endings with neurotransmitter function in single neurons. *Proceedings of the National Academy of Sciences* 73 (November): 4220–4224.

Reichardt, Louis F., and Paul H. Patterson. 1977. Neurotransmitter synthesis and uptake by isolated sympathetic neurons in microcultures. *Nature* 270 (November 10): 147–151.

Walicke, Patricia A., Robert B. Campenot and Paul H. Patterson. 1977. Determination of transmitter function by neuronal activity. *Proceedings of the National Academy of Sciences* 74 (December): 5767–5771.

Bunge, Richard P., Mary Johnson and C. David Ross. 1978. Nature and nurture in development of the autonomic neuron. *Science* 199 (March 31): 1409–1416.

Doupe, A. J., P. H. Patterson and S. C. Landis. 1985. Small intensely fluorescent cells in culture: Role of glucocorticoids and growth factors in their development and interconversions with other neural crest derivatives. *Journal of Neuroscience* 5:2143–2160.

Kessler, J. A. 1985. Differential regulation of peptide and catecholamine characteristics in cultured sympathetic neurons. *Neuroscience* 15:827–839.

Gallo, V., A. Kingsbury, R. Balázes and O. S. Jørgensen. 1987. The role of depolarization in the survival and differentiation of cerebellar granule cells in culture. *Journal of Neuroscience* 7:2203–2213.

Liles, W. C., and N. M. Nathanson. 1987. Regulation of muscarinic acetylcholine receptor number in cultured neuronal cells by chronic membrane depolarization. *Journal of Neuroscience* 8:2556–2563.

Patterson, P. H. 1987. The molecular basis of phenotypic choices in the sympathoadrenal lineage. *Annals of the New York Academy of Sciences* 93:20–23.

7. GABAergic Neurons

Caldwell, J. H., N. W. Daw and H. J. Wyatt. 1978. Effects of picrotoxin and strychnine on rabbit retinal ganglion cells: Lateral interactions for cells with more complex receptive fields. *Journal of Physiology* 276:277–298.

Gottlieb, David I., Yen-Chung Chang and James E. Schwob. 1986. Monoclonal antibodies to glutamic acid decarboxylase. *Proceedings of the National Academy of Sciences* 83 (November): 8808–8812.

Schofield, Peter R., Mark G. Darlison, Norihisa Fujita, David R. Burt, F. Anne Stephenson, Henry Rodriguez, Lucy M. Rhee, J. Ramachandran, Vincenzine Reale, Thora A. Glencorse, Peter H. Seeburg and Erica A. Barnard. 1987. Sequence and functional expression of the GABA$_A$ receptor shows a ligand-gated receptor superfamily. *Nature* 328 (July 16): 221–227.

8. Neuropeptides

Bloom, Floyd E., ed. 1980. *Peptides: Integrators of cell and tissue function.* Raven Press.

Hökfelt, Tomas, Olle Johansson, Åke Ljungdahl, Jan M. Lundberg and Marianne Schultzberg. 1980. Peptidergic neurones. *Nature* (April 10): 515–521.

Snyder, Solomon H. 1980. Brain peptides as neurotransmitters. *Science* (August 29): 976–983.

Chan, S. J., V. Episkopou, S. Zeitlin, S. K. Karathanasis, A. MacKrell, D. F. Steiner and A. Efstratidis. 1984. Guinea pig preproinsulin gene: An evolutionary compromise? *Proceedings of the National Academy of Sciences* 81:5046–5050.

Kastin, A. J., and J. E. Zadina. 1986. Multi-independent actions of peptides in the brain: LHRH, MIF-1 and CRF. *American Zoology.*

Lynch, D. R., and S. H. Snyder. 1986. Neuropeptides: Multiple molecular forms, metabolic pathways, and receptors. *Annual Review of Biochemistry* 55:773–799.

Schwartz, J. P., and E. Costa. 1986. Hybridization approaches to the study of neuropeptides. *Annual Review of Neuroscience* 9:277–304.

9. The Functional Architecture of the Retina

Ramón Y Cajal, Santiago. 1972. *The structure of the retina.* Charles C. Thomas.

Wassle, H., L. Peichl and B. B. Boycott. 1981. Dendritic territories of cat retinal ganglion cells. *Nature* 292 (July 23): 344–345.

Tauchi, M., and R. H. Masland. 1984. The cholinergic neurons in the rabbit retina. *Proceedings of the Royal Society of London, Series B* 223 (November 22): 101–119.

1986. The retina—from molecules to networks. *Trends in Neuroscience* 9 (May).

10. Transplantation in the Central Nervous System

Wallace, Robert B., and Gopal D. Das, eds. 1983. *Neural tissue transplantation research.* Springer-Verlag.

Björklund, Anders, and Ulf Stenevi, eds. 1985. *Neural grafting in the mammalian CNS.* Elsevier Science Publishers.

Fine, Alan, S. B. Dunnett, A. Björklund and S. D. Iversen. 1985. Cholinergic ventral forebrain grafts into the neocortex improve passive avoidance memory in a rat model of Alzheimer disease. *Proceedings of the National Academy of Sciences* 82 (August): 5227–5230.

Fine, R. E., and J. B. Rubin. 1988. Specific trophic factor-receptor interactions: Key selective elements in brain development and "regeneration." *Journal of the American Geriatric Society* 36:457–466.

Zager, E. L., and P. M. Black. 1988. Neural transplantation. *Surgical Neurology* 29:350–366.

INDEX

Page numbers in *italics* indicate illustrations.